Cambridge Studies in Biotechnology

Editors: Sir James Baddiley, N. H. Carey, J. F. Davidson,
I. J. Higgins, W. G. Potter

1   The biotechnology of malting and brewing

Other titles in this series

The biotechnology of malting and brewing

J. S. HOUGH

Director of the British School of Malting and Brewing
The University of Birmingham

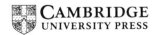

CAMBRIDGE
UNIVERSITY PRESS

PUBLISHED BY THE PRESS SYNDICATE OF THE UNIVERSITY OF CAMBRIDGE
The Pitt Building, Trumpington Street, Cambridge CB2 1RP, United Kingdom

CAMBRIDGE UNIVERSITY PRESS
The Edinburgh Building, Cambridge CB2 2RU, UK http://www.cup.cam.ac.uk
40 West 20th Street, New York, NY 10011–4211, USA http://www.cup.org
10 Stamford Road, Oakleigh, Melbourne 3166, Australia

© Cambridge University Press 1985

First published 1985
First paperback edition 1991
Reprinted 1994, 1996, 1998

Printed in the United Kingdom at the University Press, Cambridge

A catalogue record for this book is available from the British Library

ISBN 0 521 39553 4 paperback

UP

To my wife

Contents

Preface

Biotechnology has been defined as 'the application of biological organisms, systems or processes to manufacturing and service industries'. Malting and brewing are industries that exemplify traditional biotechnology, based on crafts that have been refined over thousands of years and involving, for instance, the exploitation of barley germination and yeast fermentation. It therefore seems appropriate that a series of volumes devoted to biotechnology should include one covering malting and brewing.

Much of the volume deals exclusively with malting and brewing but opportunities have been taken to describe the wider implications in agriculture and other technologies. There is therefore information on barley and hop production, the use of industrial enzymes, waste products of brewing, maize technology and the treatment of water and effluent. Modern developments in biotechnology as applied to malting and brewing also receive mention, such as genetical-manipulation techniques for improvement of malting barley and brewers' yeast. The parallels between malting and brewing and the production of beverages such as wine, cider and whiskey are briefly drawn. Reference is also made to the wide biotechnological significance of bacteria that commonly contaminate beer and breweries (or at least to their close relatives).

It is not the intention of this volume to be comprehensive in its detail of technical steps used by maltsters and brewers, or even by home brewers. Within a short text, this is not possible; the accent is instead far more on the scientific principles involved. This means that the text is directed particularly at those interested in industrial biochemistry and microbiology and, of course, in aspects of biotechnology. It should be suitable for teachers of biology and chemistry, undergraduates in appropriate disciplines and possibly sixth form students.

I wish to acknowledge the help that I have received from the staff of the Biochemistry Department of the University of Birmingham, particularly my colleagues Dr D. E. Briggs and Dr T. W. Young and from Mrs P. Hill, Mrs S. Williams, Mr J. Redfern and Mr A. Wadeson.

The kind permission of Associated Book Publishers (Chapman & Hall), London is acknowledged to reproduce figures from *Malting and Brewing Science* (1982) by J. S. Hough, D. E. Briggs, R. Stevens and

T. W. Young appearing in the present volume as 5.2–5.5, 5.7–5.8, 6.1,
6.12, 6.15, 7.1–7.5, 7.7, 8.4–8.6, 8.9–8.11, 9.1, 9.5, 9.10–9.11. My thanks
are extended to Mr J. Redfern for the photographs featuring as 2.1 (*b*),
2.5 and 7.8, and the permission of Mr A. A. James of Swan Brewery,
Perth, W. Australia for the photograph appearing as 4.1. The following
figures are based on information provided by a number of sources,
namely 5.1 partly based on drawings of Robert Morton D. G Ltd,
Burton-on-Trent; 6.11 from G. W. G. Montgomery; 6.13 from Anton
Steinecker Maschinenfabrik GmbH of Freising; 6.14 partly based on a
figure appearing in the *Practical Brewer*, published by the Master
Brewers' Association of the Americas; 7.6 based on information
provided by Dr T. W. Young; 9.12 partly based on information
provided by Mr A. Duckworth; 9.13 is based on material published by
Dr D. G. W. Brown and Dr J. F. Clapperton in the *Journal of the
Institute of Brewing*, 1978, 318.

The following tables are based on information provided or published
by the authorities stated: 1.1 (Brewers' Society, London); 1.2
(Maltsters' Association of Great Britain); 3.2 (Enari, T-M, European
Brewery Convention 1981, 69–80); 4.3 (World Health Organisation);
5.2 (work of Dr R. D. Hall); 5.3 (Professor R. H. Hopkins & Dr
B. Krause also Dr P. Kolbach & Dr G. W. Haase); 5.7 (Dr
D. Howling; 5.8 (Brewers' Grain Marketing Limited, Burton-on-Trent);
6.2 (Dr R. A. Neave and the Hops Marketing Board Limited); 6.3
(*Malting and Brewing Science*); 6.4 (from publications of Dr
J. R. Hudson and Dr D. R. J. Laws; 7.1 (Dr I. Campbell); 7.2
(R. W. Ricketts); 9.1 (Dr T. W. Young) and 9.2 (Dr J. C. Boudreau).

Abbreviations

Number	M	million
Temperature	°C	degrees Celsius
Weights	pg	picogram (10^{-12} g)
	ng	nanogram (10^{-9} g)
	μg	microgram (10^{-6} g)
	mg	milligram (10^{-3} g)
	g	gram
	kg	kilogram (10^3 g)
	Mg	megagram (10^6 g)
	tonne	megagram (10^6 g)
Volume	ml	millilitre (10^{-3} l)
	hl	hectolitre (10^2 l)
	m³	cubic metre (10^3 l)
	l	litre
Length	nm	nanometre (10^{-9} m)
	μm	micrometre or micron (10^{-6} m)
	mm	millimetre (10^{-3} m)
	cm	centimetre (10^{-2} m)
	m	metre
	km	kilometre (10^3 m)
Area	ha	hectare
Percentages	% w/v	g solute per 100 ml solvent
	% v/v	ml of component per 100 ml total
	% w/w	g of component per 100 g total
Energy	kJ	kilojoule (10^3 joule)
	MJ	megajoule (10^6 joule)
	cal	calorie
	kcal	kilocalorie (10^3 cal)
Pressure	mbar	millibar
	bar	bar
Time	s	second
	min	minute
	h	hour
Gravity	SG	specific gravity
	OG	original gravity
Effluent	SS	suspended solids (mg l^{-1})
	COD	chemical oxidation demand (mg l^{-1})

Cleaning	CIP	Cleaning-in-place
Chemical	R	radical
Money	$	US dollar
	£	pound sterling
Concentration	ppm	parts per million (usually w/v)
	ppb	parts per 10^9 (usually w/v)

1   Introduction

The mystery of brewing

The art of producing beers and wines has developed over 5000–8000 years. There must have been several independent discoveries that fermented beverages arose from exposing fruit juice or cereal extracts to the air. The explanations for the fermentations were not available until the nineteenth century but that did not impede steady improvement in manufacturing techniques. During the height of the Egyptian and Babylonian civilisations some 4300 years ago, the details of brewing were well illustrated; during Greek, and later Roman, domination wine became an important item of international commerce. The beverages were attractive, particularly for those individuals who enjoyed few pleasures, in that they produced alcoholic euphoria. Other advantages not appreciated at the time included the rendering of water of dubious microbiological quality relatively safe because of the low pH of the product and its alcoholic content. Particularly when yeast was present, the beverages provided vitamins of the B complex, a bonus to their high calorific value and content of assimilable nitrogenous material.

In the Middle Ages, brewing was an art or mystery, the details of which were jealously guarded by the master brewers and their guilds.

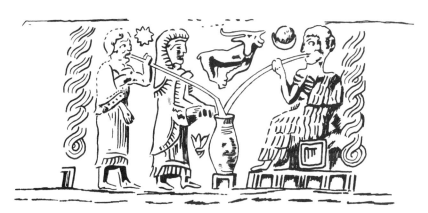

Fig. 1.1. Beer drinking in Babylonian times (2400 BC). After *100 Jahre Fakultät für Brauwesen Weihenstephan 1865–1965*, Verlag Hans Carl: Nurnberg.

And mystery it certainly was because there was virtually no appreciation of the reasons for the various processing steps, most of which, like fermentation, had been discovered by chance. Thus malting involved immersing barley in water and permitting it to sprout but the reasons for the barley becoming soft and sweet were not understood. Similarly the reasons for drying the germinated barley under relatively cool conditions were cloaked in mysticism.

Types of beer

Most beers produced until the second half of the nineteenth century were fermented with yeasts that at the end of the fermentation rose to the surface and could be skimmed off (i.e. top yeasts). Many brewers early in the history of brewing had probably failed to realise the value of the skimmings and had discarded them. Fermentation of succeeding batches had then to rely on yeast which contaminated unwashed vessels, implements and raw materials. But unhygienic conditions also permitted the incursion of unwanted yeasts and bacteria that produced unwanted flavours and hazes. For these reasons, there must until recent times have been great batch-to-batch variation and many beers would have been vinegary due to infections by acetic acid bacteria.

Hops were introduced into Britain from Flanders in the sixteenth century by Flemish immigrants. Competition and conflict arose between those producing the traditional unhopped ale and the brewers making the new 'beer'. Nowadays beer is a generic expression encompassing what we term ale, a hopped beverage made with top yeasts, together with those hopped malt beverages which are fermented with bottom yeasts. Bottom yeasts are those which, at the end of fermentation, sink in the vessels; they were first employed in Bavaria. Compared with most top yeasts they produced a superior product. It is not surprising therefore that, when the Bavarians released them to other regions, these yeasts gradually replaced top yeasts in most parts of the world. They are used for producing beers called 'lagers', after the German word meaning storage or cellaring.

Recent history of brewing

Brewing grew apace with improved roads, canals and railways. This was especially true of the larger breweries which were able to sustain an expanding national and even international market. This trade left its mark on beers called 'India Pale Ale', 'Russian Stout' and 'Export'. The breweries which were most successful were those with natural water supplies appropriate to the beers they were producing. Thus, Pilsen gave its name to pale European lagers either as 'Pils' or 'Pilsner'. Any water can now be modified to match that of Burton-on-Trent or Pilsen. The large breweries now have other problems with their water: is it suitable for modern steam-raising equipment and automatic cleaning systems and is there opportunity for discharging the large volumes of watery effluent from the brewery into the municipal drains?

Breweries originally used manpower or water power for driving equipment but the advent of steam engines permitted almost unfettered expansion of the brewery and of the size of equipment. The main problem for breweries was that certain processes in malting and brewing required cool conditions. Malting and brewing were therefore restricted in temperate countries to the autumn, winter and spring and were unsuitable for tropical countries. About the beginning of the twentieth century, refrigeration equipment based on ammonia compressors became available. This has permitted malting and brewing to be carried out throughout the year in both temperate and tropical regions.

Organisation of the industry

Brewing is an important industry. About 9.5×10^{10} l are produced annually in the world, of which the UK contributes 6×10^9 l. Except for Denmark, Eire and the Netherlands, only a small proportion of the beer produced in a country is exported, although franchise brewing (brewing under licence) is common. Britain is unique in having vertical integration of its brewing industry, with several firms involved in

Table 1.1. *Beer production and consumption volumes in 1981 for countries producing more than 2×10^9 l*

	Production (1×10^9)	Consumption ($l\ head^{-1}$)
USA	22.7	93
Federal Republic of Germany	9.3	147
USSR	6.3	23
UK	6.2	112
Japan	4.6	39
Mexico	2.9	40
Brazil	2.4	24
Czechoslovakia	2.4	140
German Democratic Republic	2.4	138
Canada	2.3	86
France	2.2	44
Spain	2.1	55
World total	96.8	

malting, hop growing, brewing, wholesaling and retailing. As in the USA, there have been extensive amalgamations and take-overs of UK brewery companies so that the number of breweries has tended to fall markedly.

Legislation

In 1516 the Bavarian authorities introduced Beer Purity Laws (Reinheitsgebot) which restricted brewing materials to malted barley, water, hops and yeast. These laws gradually extended to the whole of Germany until, in 1918, they applied to all beers except those intended for export. They have been matched in a number of other European countries such as Norway, Greece and Switzerland. Elsewhere in the world it is usual to include in brewing materials inexpensive sources of starch or sugar such as unmalted cereals, refined potato-starch and syrups derived from sugar cane, sugar beet or cereals. Also used in brewing are small amounts of inorganic and organic materials used as preservatives (e.g. sulphur dioxide) or for preventing turbidity (e.g. papain, a proteolytic enzyme). In recent years many countries have introduced stringent controls of such additives and insist on the package label showing details of them. Controls on levels of arsenic and lead in raw materials and beers have been in force for many years. Recently restrictions on nitrosamine levels in malted barley and beers have been introduced. Nitrosamines are known to be carcinogenic in large doses to laboratory mammals but have not as yet been shown conclusively to be harmful to humans.

An outline of malting

Malt is cereal grain, usually barley, which has been germinated for a limited period of time, and then dried. The maltster is therefore concerned with accumulating stocks of suitable barley, storing them until required, steeping the grain in water and allowing the barley corns to germinate. At a time that he considers appropriate, the maltster arrests germination by drying the grain in a stream of warm air. The malted corn represents a package for the brewer that will keep stable for months, if not years. During the germination, the food store or endosperm of the corn is partly degraded by enzymes that attack cell walls, starch granules and the protein matrix. The package provided is therefore the degraded endosperm and the attendant enzymes able to complete the degradation.

When relatively cool air is used for drying, the malt is pale in colour and very rich in enzymes. With greater drying temperatures, especially early in the drying process, the malt is darker in colour and the enzymic

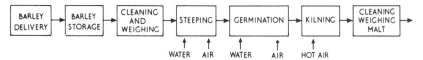

Fig. 1.2. Flow diagram of the malting process.

content is depleted. Some malts used in small amounts for colouring and flavouring have no detectable enzymic activity.

An outline of brewing

Brewing in its simplest form (Fig. 1.3) involves:

(*a*)   Crushing malted barley to form a very coarse flour called the grist.

(*b*)   Adding warm water to the grist to form a porridge-like mash. Malt enzymes are encouraged to solubilise the degraded endosperm of the ground malt.

(*c*)   Separating in a suitable vessel the aqueous extract, called wort, from the spent solids by spraying further supplies of hot water onto the mash.

(*d*)   Boiling the wort with hops. This stops enzyme action, sterilises the wort, coagulates some proteins; the hops impart distinctive flavours and aromas to the wort.

(*e*)   Clarifying, cooling and aerating the wort so that it is an ideal medium for yeast growth and fermentation.

(*f*)   Fermenting the wort with yeast so that much of the carbohydrate is converted into alcohol and carbon dioxide. Other yeast metabolites contribute to flavour and aroma.

(*g*)   Maturing and clarifying the beer. Modifying the flavour aroma and keeping qualities of the beer.

(*h*)   Packaging the beer, usually after it has been either sterile-filtered or pasteurised. Alternatively, for small packages like bottles or cans, it can be pasteurised within the package.

Beer strength

The strength of beer is usually expressed in terms of the specific gravity at the beginning of fermentation or Original Gravity (OG). For a given value however there may be varying amounts of fermentable matter; the extent to which the yeast has fermented this matter may also vary. Thus the level of alcohol present in the beer is not necessarily proportional to the OG. Few beers are below OG 1.030 because they are prone to mould infections in addition to aggregated yeast and bacterial infections. In many countries the specific gravity notation is replaced by one based on the per cent by weight of sucrose in water that has the same specific gravity as the solution being measured. Very roughly 1.008 is equivalent to 2%, 1.040 to 10% (i.e. each per cent

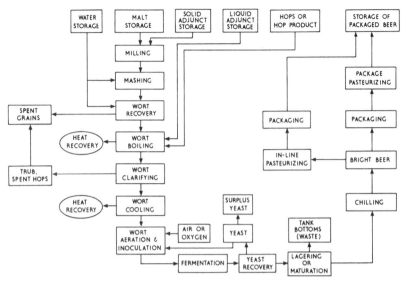

Fig. 1.3. Flow diagram of the brewing process.

sucrose accounts for 0.004). These percentage values are usually given as °Balling or in the more accurate °Plato.

Classification of beers

Beers made from malted barley, with or without carbohydrate adjuncts water, hops and yeast.

(a)   Ales – fermented with a top-fermentation yeast
  (i)   Pale ales (OG 1032–48) – made mainly from pale malts and strongly hopped, usually little sweetness, includes Kolsch beer from Cologne and district
  (ii)   Bitter (OG 1032–48) – the term used for draught pale ales
  (iii) Brown ales (OG 1032–48) – made with malts that give a deeply coloured beer, usually sweeter and less hopped than pale ales
  (iv)   Mild (OG 1032–40) – usually the draught equivalent of brown ales, however some areas have pale coloured mild.
  (v)   Stout (OG 1032–55) – the darkest ales but some are intensely bitter with no sweetness while others are sweet
  (vi)   Barley wine (OG 1065–1100) – usually a very strong pale ale
(b)   Lagers – fermented with bottom yeast (untergärige)
  (i)   Pale (Hell or Pilsner) (OG 1032–48) – made with pale malt, no sweetness, distinctive hop flavour and aroma
  (ii)   Dark (Dunkel) (OG 1042–55) – made with darker malts, sometimes slightly sweet and stronger than the pale
  (iii) Märzen, Bock (OG 1050–5) – special strong beers, traditionally made at certain times of the year

(*c*)   Weissbier, Weizenbier (OG 1028–34) – made with a mixture of malted barley and malted wheat, worts boiled but unhopped, fermented with bottom yeast; usually drunk with lemon slices or fruit juice

(*d*)   African native beers – made with malted sorghum, millets, plus in some cases malted barley; worts unboiled and unhopped; served unclarified and actively fermenting

2   Barley – the key material

Why barley?

Several cereals can be satisfactorily malted but barley usually gives least technical difficulty. Maize is rarely, if ever, malted because its fat becomes rancid. Wheat is malted on a commercial scale, particularly for certain special breads but microbial growth on the surface of the corn during germination may cause problems. For the production of African native beers, a variety of cereals (especially sorghum) are malted. Nevertheless, it is the flavour of beer made from malted barley rather than other materials that has been appreciated over the years by most of the world. Furthermore the barley used for brewing malts has a high starch content and it is this material that yields the fermentable extract. Protein is also present and there is usually more than sufficient to provide the amino acids needed for yeast growth and the nitrogenous material important in forming beer foam.

Many varieties of barley are sown. They may differ not only in the form of the whole plant or the appearance of the ear, but also in physiological features. Thus some have been bred for autumn/winter sowing in temperate climates while others are adapted to spring sowing. Varieties are available that show dormancy of the corns. This is advantageous if the mature ear becomes damp before harvesting so that conditions are right for the corns to germinate while still in the ear. It is disadvantageous if it prevents the maltster from germinating the corns

Table 2.1. *Barley production in 1981 (million tonnes)*

Continental distribution		Principal producers	
Africa	3.2	USSR	43.0
Asia	17.2	Canada	13.4
Australasia	3.6	USA	10.4
Europe	66.3	France	10.2
North America	24.4	UK	10.1
South America	0.8		
USSR	43.0		
World total	158.5		87.1

without complex and lengthy treatment. Quite apart from the genetic traits of the barley, the effects of climate and soil have to be considered. In the northern hemisphere, barley will grow well from the Scandinavian countries south to the African countries which border the Mediterranean. It will also grow in the tropical highlands such as in Kenya. The main areas of production in the world are the USSR, Canada, USA, France and the UK (Table 2.1).

Development of the plant

In the field, the corn germinates (providing that it is not dormant) when it finds sufficient water and oxygen and the temperature is above 5 °C. The first sign of germination is the appearance of a small white spike protruding from the corn; this is actually a sheath which protects five seminal rootlets within (Fig. 2.1a, b). When the sheath splits, the rootlets ramify the soil particles, develop root hairs and take up water and mineral salts. Soon after, the leaf sheath (coleoptile) breaks out near the end of the corn away from the rootlets and extends rapidly to the soil surface. The coleoptile then splits, revealing the first true leaf. Each leaf arises at successive joints (nodes) on the stem and it is convenient to refer to the physiological age of the plant by the number of leaves that have emerged (Fig. 2.2). This provides a guide in the application of insecticidal and fungicidal sprays, as well as fertilisers.

It is a characteristic of many barley varieties that secondary shoots or tillers arise from the base of the primary stem. Each tiller becomes equivalent to the primary stem in bearing a flowering head. Before flowering occurs, however, the stems elongate by extending between each node. The flowering head (inflorescence) is finally revealed as the uppermost leaves unroll. During this development above ground, the original (seminal) roots branch and extend. The root system is supplemented by adventitious roots developing at the bases of the various shoots. This extension of the system allows the plant to take up water and mineral salts from a wide area, to a maximum depth of 2 m, in addition to providing a formidable anchor.

Modern varieties of barley have relatively short stems (60–90 cm). The winter barleys are usually checked in their growth during the colder months and extend in length in the summer. Each flowering head has an axis with short internodes (Fig. 2.2). From a node arises three simple flowers, grouped on one side of the stem. At the next node, the grouping is on the opposite side. Therefore, looking vertically down on the flower axis, six rows of flowers should be apparent (Fig. 2.3). However, while in some varieties all the flowers are fertile, in other varieties only the central flower of the three will form a fruit. Thus we can distinguish between 6-row and 2-row barleys. In the UK it is rare

(*a*)

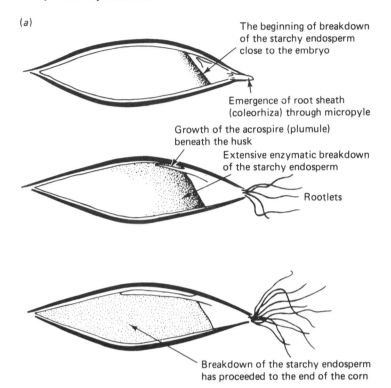

The beginning of breakdown
of the starchy endosperm
close to the embryo

Emergence of root sheath
(coleorhiza) through micropyle

Growth of the acrospire (plumule)
beneath the husk

Extensive enzymatic breakdown
of the starchy endosperm

Rootlets

Breakdown of the starchy endosperm
has proceeded to the end of the corn

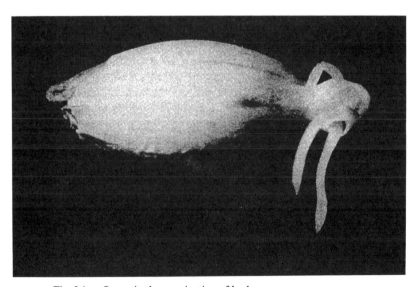

Fig. 2.1. *a.* Stages in the germination of barley.
b. A germinating barley corn. The embryo has developed rootlets that have
emerged from the protective layers.

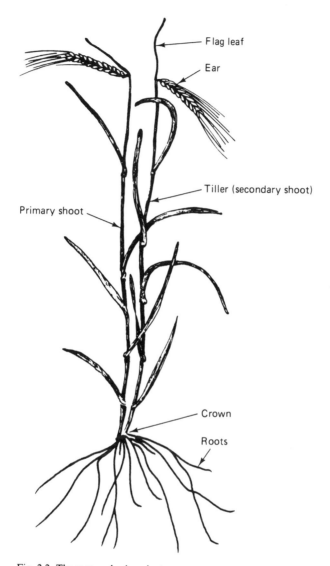

Fig. 2.2. The mature barley plant.

to grow 6-row varieties for malting but in the USA both 2-row and 6-row barleys are grown for malting. With the 6-row, the fruits or corns that develop have less space for development than with 2-row. Hence the central flower tends to produce a normal corn but the two lateral flowers (which are sterile in 2-row varieties) form rather twisted, thin corns.

Barley is apparently adapted to wind pollination but usually less than

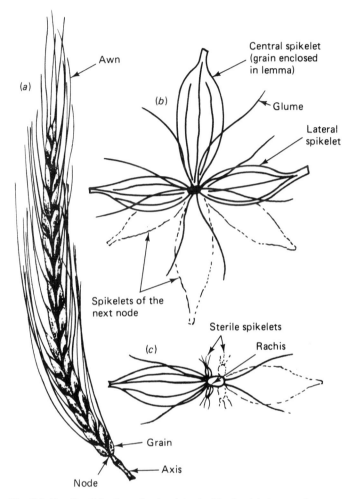

Fig. 2.3. Details of the flowering head (ear) of barley (*a*) the ear of a two-rowed barley, (*b*) a six-rowed barley ear seen from above, and (*c*) a two-rowed barley ear seen from above. The dotted outline represents the florets attached at the next node or joint.

1% are cross-pollinated. The high incidence of self-pollination has a profound effect on breeding techniques and on the genetic constitution of the corns in the field. When the haploid egg in the ovule fuses with a nucleus from the pollen tube, cell division and differentiation of the diploid cell leads to the formation of the new embryo plant. A second pollen tube nucleus fuses with a diploid cell in the ovule to yield triploid tissue which serves as the food store of the corn (the endosperm). To protect and encase both the embryo and endosperm, the seed and fruit walls fuse and, in most cases, fuse also with the two scale-like bracts of the flower. This protective layer is called the husk. In some varieties, one of the flower bracts is extended into a spear or awn. Alternatively, it may be folded into a hood-like appendage.

The barley corn

Figure 2.4 and 2.5 show the barley corn in longitudinal and transverse section. The bracts called the lemma and palea are shown, the former extended into an awn. At their base is the former attachment of the flower to the mother plant and close to it is a region called the micropyle through which air and water can permeate to the embryo plant. The embryo is arranged mainly on the rounded or dorsal side of the corn. Its root sheath is close to the micropyle so that it can readily penetrate through this region when germination commences. In contrast the embryonic shoot points toward the distal end of the corn. Separating the embryo from its food store or endosperm is a shield-shaped structure called the scutellum, regarded by some as the seed-leaf of this monocotyledonous plant. The bulk of the endosperm is made up of large non-living cells, each of which is packed with large

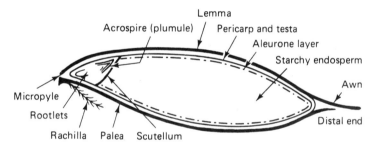

Fig. 2.4. Longitudinal (vertical) section through a barley corn.

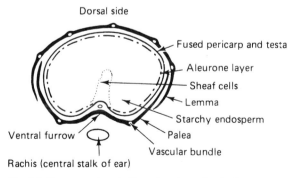

Fig. 2.5. Transverse (vertical) section through a barley corn.

and small starch grains. A mantle of protein invests the starch grains and some fat is also present. The thin cell walls mainly comprise hemicellulose and glucan gums. On the periphery of the endosperm is a layer of small living cells which are rich in protein but free of starch grains; this is called the aleurone layer. This region which is three cells thick, does not extend over the scutellum; there its place is taken by a layer of crushed cells devoid of contents.

The husk and fruit-coat are protective in function. They also ensure, by capillarity, that water is distributed effectively over the surface of corn. This water can then penetrate to the embryo, partly by the micropyle and partly by any chance cracks in the husk. The seed-coat, fused to the fruit-coat, is selectively permeable. It prevents not only the escape of sugars and amino acids from the corn, but also the entry of microorganisms. Chance cracks through these layers permit loss of nutrients, microbial growth in the tissues and loss of mechanical strength. In extreme cases they may even prevent the embryo from germinating. The scutellum has a secretory function, permitting release of hydrolytic enzymes from the embryo into the starchy endosperm. Enzymic degradation of protein, starch and cell walls provides soluble food in the form of amino acids and sugars that diffuse into the embryo and sustain its growth.

The aleurone layer has also a secretory function but, until germination is under way, its enzyme complement is mainly restricted to the carbohydrase, amylase. During its early growth, the embryo releases the plant hormone gibberellin which, in its turn, triggers the aleurone layer to increase its range of enzymes. This it does either by activating enzyme precursors or by initiating the full biosynthesis of the enzymes. As the enzymes are secreted from the scutellum and aleurone, they attack the starchy endosperm progressively towards the distal end of the corn. Although the protein, starch and cell wall material are only partly degraded, the corn nevertheless becomes noticeably softer in texture and the contents progressively sweeter in taste. The maltster calls these changes 'modification'.

The farmers' requirements

In Britain, just less than 20% of the barley grown is used for malting (Table 2.2). The rest is mainly used for animal feed. It might be thought therefore that certain barley varieties would be grown for animal feed where a high content of protein is required, and other varieties selected for malting where a high content of starch is demanded. This is only partly true. Barley varieties are bred which will give protein-rich corns when grown under a regime of high nitrogen fertilisers but it is an added advantage if such varieties will malt well and give starch-rich

Table 2.2. *Use of barley in the UK (thousand tonnes)*

	Year		
	1971/2	1976/7	1981/2
Malting	1276	1396	1432
Animal feed	7433	6252	4837

The UK Cereals Market, Ministry of Agriculture, Food and Fisheries.

corns under a different fertiliser treatment. This is because a malting barley variety normally gives a poorer yield in terms of tonne per hectare than a feed barley variety. The maltster will not pay the full economic premium for the malting variety but instead uses feed barley varieties that are known to malt well. He selects from these the batches that are relatively rich in starch and low in protein.

The main requirement for the farmer is then high yield per hectare possible by tillering. In order to have a reasonable chance of this, the barley must not only have the genetic constitution to yield well under ideal conditions, it must also be resistant to the common diseases of barley (e.g. mildew and rust). To combat adverse weather conditions, the flowering stems must be short and stiff. If they are layed to the ground by wind or rain or trampling, they should have some ability to rise from this lodged (flattened) condition. Some old varieties were unsuitable for modern mechanical harvesting, for instance the fruiting heads shattered so that the corns were scattered over the ground. Finally, the farmer who can harvest early tends to have advantages in selling the grain at a higher price and in this connection, winter-sown varieties tend to be earlier harvested than spring-sown.

The maltsters' requirements

The maltster has the advantage in the UK that extensive trials are carried out on each barley variety by the National Institute of Agricultural Botany and the ability of that barley to malt is graded. What the maltster needs first and foremost is a barley which will germinate evenly and easily. Even or synchronous germination is unlikely to occur unless the corns are of uniform size. This is because, among other things, large corns take up moisture at a slower rate relative to their weight than small corns. Another consideration is that the barley to be malted must not have germinated before harvesting, nor must any of the corns be dead due to unsatisfactory drying of the grain after harvest. What the maltster needs is more than 98% of the corns showing the emergence of the root sheath after steeping. Such barley is said to have 'chitted'.

Another requirement already mentioned is a relatively low protein level, say 9.5–11.5%. Usually it is the total nitrogen content of the grains which is measured, say 1.55–1.85%. (It is conventional, but not usually strictly accurate, that the nitrogen content $\times$ 6.25 is equal to the protein content.) The argument that less protein means more starch can also be applied to the husk. Hence the maltster wants low protein and low husk in his barleys. Recently attention has been paid to low polyphenol (or tannin) content. This has little influence on starch levels but does influence the storage life of the beer eventually produced.

The maltster also wants a barley which, when malted, will perform well in the brewing process. It should have a satisfactory enzyme complement so that mashing presents no problem. The wort must separate easily from the spent grain and, in this connection, the barley should have a low content of certain gummy carbohydrates called β glucans. It will thus be appreciated that selecting new varieties of malting barley is difficult.

The maltsters' requirements do not end here; there are batches that have to be rejected for other reasons, such as mould contamination or infestation with insects or rodents.

Two-row and six-row barleys

In the USA, 6-row barleys exclusively were malted in the past. The barleys yielded well and malted well but their protein content was usually high, say 11.5–12.5. One advantage of higher protein contents is that there tends to be a greater enzyme complement. Thus 6-row barleys produced a malt with a lower starch content but a greater enzyme content. The level of enzymes was such that the brewer could mix equal weights of malt and cereal starch and still produce his wort satisfactorily. Further, such malts were ideal for other industrial applications needing a high enzyme complement rather than the extractable solids (e.g. in baking, desizing of cloth or grain-whiskey manufacture.

More recently in the USA, 2-row barleys have become important. They have on average larger, more uniform corns and contain more starch than 6-rowed barleys. Their enzyme level may be lower but nevertheless in modern varieties is more than adequate for an equal mix with cereal starch.

Why then have 6-rowed barleys not been used for malting in the UK? Certainly 6-rowed barleys are imported from North America for making distillers' malt. The answer is that the 6-rowed strains have been rejected because of the lack of uniformity of their corns, their high protein, high husk and low starch levels. Yet some 50 years ago, North American 6-rowed malts were used in UK breweries, partly because of their high enzymic content and partly because the husks improved the filtering qualities of the mash bed (wetted ground malt within a mash tun).

Barley breeding

In most cases, new barley varieties have arisen by artificially crossing one existing variety with another. The object is to combine together in one plant advantageous traits, such as disease resistance and early ripening, found in different varieties. Sometimes one of the parents of the cross will be subjected to artificial mutation. In other cases, the breeder will use primitive or even wild strains in order to obtain, for instance, resistance to the barley rust fungi.

The breeder must prevent the barley plants from self-pollinating. He therefore designates one plant as the 'mother' and from this he removes all the stamens before they have matured. He then transfers pollen from the 'father' plant to the stigmas of the mother, using a brush. The flowering head of the mother is then protected with a bag to prevent accidental cross-pollination by wind or insects. From this cross will arise a few hybrid seeds which are carefully germinated.

The hybrid barley plants which develop are carefully monitored at every stage. If satisfactory, they may be artificially crossed again or be allowed to self-pollinate naturally. At each generation, the plants are carefully selected and, of course, the number of corns available for study becomes larger. It is not normally until the ninth generation that there is enough seed corn to sell to farmers. By this time its characters will be well described. However its success on each soil type and microclimate will not be known. It therefore takes many years to produce a new variety, a process that can only be hastened by flying the precious corn each autumn for spring sowing in suitable ground in the opposite hemisphere of the world. With each generation, the heterozygosity of the original hybrid is gradually lost and some reselection may be needed. Varieties thus have limited life and even a really successful variety is superseded by an improved one after 3–10 years.

To indicate the way in which barley breeding may go, a barley has been developed in which the biosynthesis of a group of tannins has been blocked. Compounds of this group are called anthocyanogens and are important to the keeping qualities of beer. They react with proteins to form complexes that will gradually polymerise until the material becomes insoluble and makes the beer hazy. By keeping the level of anthocyanogens low, these barleys offer a novel method of combatting haze. The barley concerned is a mutant form of the variety *Foma* called *ant-13*. It can be malted readily and the keeping qualities of the beers produced are in direct relation with the proportion of the ant-13 malt used. At the present there are some snags because the yield of the barley in the field tends to be low, particularly if the barley is infested by powdery mildew fungus. There are several improvements to the system that have to be made but no reason why such barleys should not be available in quantity in a few years' time.

Barley brewing

Some breweries use a mixture of malted and unmalted barley for brewing. With less than 30% raw barley, the enzymes of the malt may suffice to degrade the starch, protein and cell walls. It is usual however with barley brewing to supplement the malt enzymes with industrial enzymes of microbial origin, such as β glucanase, a amylase and neutral protease from *Bacillus subtilis*. The barley is selected for large corn size, low protein and low moisture content. It is either dry milled, or wet milled after steeping, mixed with malt and industrial enzymes, then subjected to temperature-programmed mashing before wort recovery. Although the process is claimed to be less expensive than conventional wort production (because barley is cheaper than malt) it has not proved popular for several reasons, such as milling problems, viscosity difficulties, flavour differences and reluctance to have barley and industrial enzymes published as ingredients of beer. The proteolytic enzymes of germinating barley and finished malt produce a free amino acid mixture, characterised by having a high proportion of the imino acid proline which is not used by brewing yeast during fermentation. (See p. 27) Beer made by barley brewing can therefore be discriminated by its lower content of proline because the protein of the unmalted barley is less easily degraded than the protein of malted barley.

3 Malt – a package of enzymes and food substances

Storing barley

Barley is most stable when it is dry and cool. If barley has been harvested by a combine harvester at moisture contents above 15%, it is usually dried either at the farm or at the maltings. The drying process has to be carried out in such a way that the embryonic plant in each corn remains viable. Too high a temperature, therefore, is avoided and speeding up of the drying must be based on increased air flow as well as additional heating. In a typical 2 h drying, the drying air may start at 54 °C and reach 66 °C, but the grain temperature never exceeds 52 °C. Heating usually has another desirable effect, that of reducing the time needed before dormancy ends. A typical treatment is to dry to 12% moisture and then to store at 25 °C for 7–14 days. It is then usual to permit the temperature to fall to 15 °C while carrying out cleaning and grading of corn size. Movement of the grain from one silo to another also helps to make the temperature of a large mass of grain uniform and to introduce oxygen to maintain the respiration of the embryos.

Moist grain is readily attacked by insect pests and spoilage fungi, especially if the temperature is in excess of 15 °C. When they do establish themselves, the metabolism of the insects or fungi gives rise to water and to increased local temperature. This encourages further spread of the infestation. Under extreme conditions, the rise in temperature may even lead to the grain catching fire. It is therefore good practice to have in each silo several temperature probes. Any significant change in temperature can be detected and action taken to prevent serious damage.

The insects that are commonly encountered in maltings are the saw-toothed grain beetle, the grain weevil and the flat grain beetle. There are some such as the Khapra beetle that can breed in grain at very low moisture contents, even in finished malt with 2% moisture. Many microorganisms grow on barley corns, including moulds, yeasts and bacteria. Of these, the most important tend to be filamentous fungi such as *Aspergillus*. There is a very high level of infestation if the barley is subjected to wet conditions when mature, that is if the grain is 'weathered'. Such fungi however are displaced during storage by other fungi, often closely related, called 'storage fungi'. There is particular

19

concern that barley is not contaminated by fungi such as *Aspergillus fumigatus* whose spores cause lung damage (farmer's lung). Also to be avoided are those fungi that produce aflotoxins – happily they are rare – and the ergot fungus *Claviceps purpurea* that develops, on the barley grains, black fruiting bodies which are rich in the poison ergotamine.

Selection of barley

Barley arrives at the maltings in large road trucks or railway cars. It is necessary to judge the quality of the barley quickly, in most instances. The maltster inspects visually to see whether the grain is of uniform size, free of unwanted material such as weed seeds, broken corns and rodent droppings. Barley which has been badly infested by microorganisms gives a characteristic odour which the maltster can readily detect. Other tests are carried out in the laboratory. These include analysis of moisture content, viability of the embryos and the nitrogen content of the grain. In large maltings, the moisture measurement is estimated by electrical conductivity or by an infrared reflectance spectrometer. The protein content is measured either by converting it to ammonium sulphate and titrating the ammonia or by dye-binding of the protein or, again, by the infrared reflectance spectrometer. Finally the viability of the embryos may be estimated by cutting the grains longitudinally and soaking them in a tetrazolium salt. Living embryos have active dehydrogenase enzymes that reduce the salt to a red formazan dye which stains the embryos. This rapid test is usually confirmed by small-scale germination tests.

There are two forms of dormancy in barley – profound dormancy and water-sensitivity. Profound dormancy refers to embryos of the barley which are temporarily unable to germinate. The condition is common after the fruiting head has matured in cool, damp conditions; it prevents pre-germination of the embryos while they are still present in the fruiting head. Dormancy can be broken most conveniently by warm storage but also, in the laboratory, by peeling off the husk, fruit and seed-coats. Water-sensitivity is the condition under which barley will germinate in a minimum volume of water but fails to do so if submerged, especially if the water is not saturated with air. It can be avoided by spray-steeping or using several steeps, each of short duration, or by saturating the steep water with oxygen. Water-sensitive barleys appear to need a higher concentration of oxygen in the embryo tissues than non-sensitive barleys. Maltsters will therefore select batches of barleys that have a dormancy that is lost after a few weeks' storage. They will avoid, if they can, water-sensitive barleys or they will adjust the steeping regime to overcome the condition.

Steeping

The steeping schedule is usually optimised from results with small-scale trials (micromalting trials). Typically, a clean barley batch will be dropped from a silo into a steep tank partly filled with water at say 15 °C. Many steep tanks are vertical cylinders with conical bases (Fig. 3.1). Air is either perfused through the steep water using perforated pipes or is pulled through the water by suction. Most steep tanks constructed recently are shallow flat-bottomed vertical cylinders (Fig. 3.2); these permit more aerobic conditions to prevail in the steep water.

When first immersed, the moisture content of the grain increases rapidly but then slows down progressively. The speed is a function of the growth conditions of the barley prior to harvesting, the size of the corns, the variety of the barley and the temperature of the water. It is also influenced greatly by the amount of mechanical damage done to the corns before steeping. Indeed before steeping the maltster may, with certain batches of barley, choose deliberately to abrade the barley in a machine which scrapes the husk off each corn at the distal end (the portion furthest away from the embryo).

The steeping is interrupted after 12–24 h by draining. Each barley corn remains covered with a film of water through which oxygen from the surrounding air can readily dissolve. This condition is known as 'air-rest'. The steep water going to waste is contaminated with a certain amount of barley dust and also endosperm from damaged corns. It is therefore rich in suspended and dissolved organic matter, and is an effluent which requires treatment before it can be discharged into rivers and lakes. After a few hours air-rest, the barley is reimmersed in a

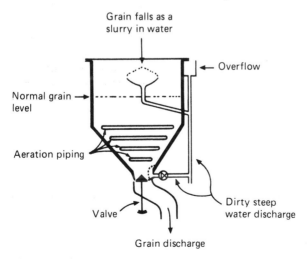

Fig. 3.1. A cylindroconical steep tank.

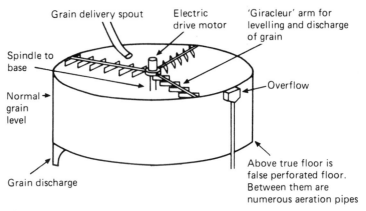

Fig. 3.2. A modern flat-bottomed steep tank.

second steep water; the alternation of steep and air-rest continues until the barley has reached about 42% moisture. By this time, it is likely that the grain has begun to chit (reveal the rootlets).

When barley is steeped, the water quickly penetrates the husk and fruit-coat, and enters the corn through or near the micropyle. The embryo takes up water quickly while the endosperm hydrates more slowly. Any cracks in the husk, fruit- and seed-coat permit more rapid moistening of the endosperm or embryo and, of course, easy escape of soluble endosperm material. This loss of material is one aspect of 'malting loss'; another component is the loss due to respiration by the embryo, consuming food reserves to yield energy, carbon dioxide and water. The respiration increases significantly when the embryo becomes active; this creates a massive oxygen demand in the steep water – hence the sparging (perfusion) of air and the air-rests during steeping. In the absence of oxygen, the embryo has some capacity to metabolise anaerobically by converting food reserves rather wastefully into energy, carbon dioxide and alcohol. As the alcohol concentration increases, it becomes progressively more toxic.

Germination

Steeping is normally completed in about 2 days; in modern malting techniques, the corns have chitted at the end of the process. They are transferred either as a slurry to germination equipment or, preferably, by 'dry' transfer (which causes less damage to the embryos). The moisture content is in the region of 42% in most cases and, during the germination phase, it will remain so.

Traditionally, steeped grain is spread onto a malting floor in an even couch of about 25 cm depth. The flooring material is impervious to water but any loss of moisture by evaporation may be made good by sprinkling water. A wooden malt shovel is used to 'turn' the batch of germinating barley. This turning action dissipates carbon dioxide produced by respiration, brings fresh air to the embryos, evens the temperature (which tends to rise because of the respiration), and prevents rootlets from matting. The speed at which the rootlets grow once they break out of the root sheath is remarkable. Temperature is maintained around 15 °C and, therefore, summer malting demands air-conditioning. A floor-malting schedule on the germination floor extends over 4–6 days. Its progress is monitored by taking regular samples for the laboratory. One simple and useful guide is to examine the growth of the embryonic shoot (variously called the coleoptile or acrospire). Usually the maltster continues germination until this structure has grown $\frac{2}{3}$ the length of the corn (Fig. 2.1). It is, of course, not visible unless the corn is broken longitudinally because it grows beneath the fruit- and seed-coats.

Modern equipment permits germination in 3–4 days and far greater depths of malt to be loaded. The most common type takes the form of a rectangular or circular box fitted with a perforated false floor (Fig. 3.3). Malt is loaded onto the false floor to a depth of 1.0–1.5 m. Water-saturated air, at about 15 °C, is blown or sucked through the bed (usually upwards). This ensures that there is oxygen available for the embryos, that carbon dioxide is swept away and that a constant temperature is maintained in the bed. In order that the rootlets do not mat together, a mechanical turner separates the germinating corns. It also helps to aerate and maintain an even temperature.

Sometimes one vessel is used for both steeping and germination, thus saving transfer of the grain. Usually, however, the steeps are immediately above the germination vessels. In some maltings, the germination vessels double up as kilns, again saving transfer. The kilning operation dries and sterilises the vessel but there are problems operating machinery at widely differing temperatures. A feature of many modern maltings is their tower construction with steeps above

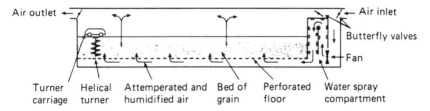

Fig. 3.3. Vertical section through a pneumatic germination box.

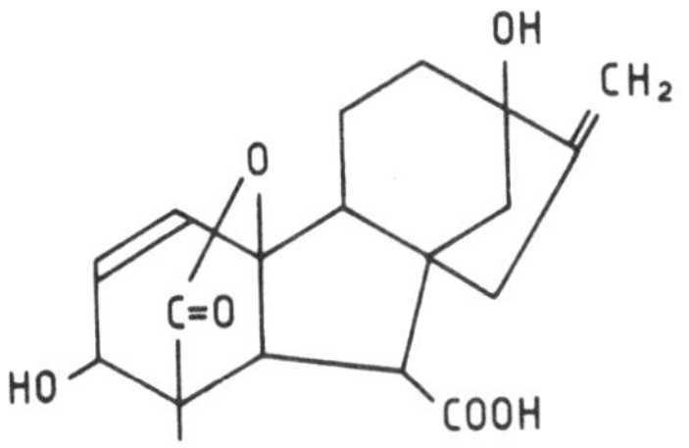

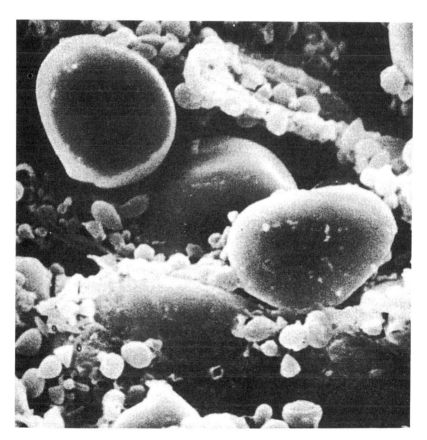

Fig. 3.4. Gibberellic acid.

Fig. 3.5. Starchy endosperm cells of malted barley viewed by electron microscopy. Large and small starch grains are visible along with a portion of cell wall.

germination vessels and kilns at the base. There can therefore be a gravity feed of grain from top to bottom.

From a physiological point of view, there is continuity between steeping and germination. The embryonic growth is initiated in steeping and because the food reserves immediately available to it are limited, it is necessary for the abundant reserves of the endosperm to be mobilised. This is achieved by the embryo or scutellum secreting enzymes to degrade the protein, starch and cell walls of the endosperm. On its own, this would be insufficient for the needs of the rapidly developing embryo. They are met by the mobilisation of the aleurone layer to produce enzymes either from complex precursors or from amino acids. The trigger for mobilisation is one or more plant hormones called gibberellins (Fig. 3.4) that are secreted by the embryo and diffuse to the aleurone. Enzyme breakdown of the endosperm therefore proceeds from the embryo end of the corn to the distal end, also from the outer regions to the inner regions. The physical weakening of the endosperm structure and the biochemical degradations are referred to as modification. Malted corns can therefore be referred to as under-modified, well-modified or over-modified, depending on how extensive is the enzymic degradation. Under-modified malt very often has a region at the distal end which completely lacks modification; it is said to have hard ends.

Biochemistry of barley germination

One of the most early physical changes of the endosperm during germination may be observed by electron microscopy. At the beginning of germination, it is difficult to see the starch grains because of a veil or investment of protein that covers them. Within a day of the start of germination this largely disappears revealing the starch grains and cell walls (Fig. 3.5). It is likely that the cell walls are attacked throughout the germination.

Proteins

Turning first to the barley proteins, it should be noted that the proteins present are not simple mixtures that can readily be characterised. Not only is there complexity before germination, the degradative processes produce an array of new, simpler compounds. A traditional but useful way of classifying barley proteins is based on solubility in various solvents (Table 3.1). Thus proteins soluble in salt solution are the relatively simple albumins and globulins; these include enzymes. The protein material which is insoluble in salt solution but soluble in warm alcohol is more complex; this is called hordein. Finally, protein

Table 3.1. *Simple classification of barley and malt proteins based on solubility*

Protein	Soluble in	Represented in barley grain as
Albumin	Water	Enzymes
Globulin	Dilute salt solutions	Enzymes
Prolamin (Hordein)	Hot 70% ethanol	Storage protein
Glutelin	Dilute alkali or acid	Structural protein

material insoluble in the warm alcohol is called glutelin. The hordein represents mainly storage protein, the nitrogenous reserve for the barley embryo, material which is degraded by proteases into simple nitrogenous compounds such as proteoses, peptones and, simplest of all, amino acids. The glutelin is mainly structural protein which, during germination, shows little change in quantity.

During germination, some of the carbohydrate is respired and therefore, as a percentage of the entire corn, the proteins and related compounds appear to increase. However some of the simpler nitrogenous compounds are used to build up the proteins of the rootlets. After kilning, the rootlets are removed from the corns so that the protein content appears to fall. One important parameter to both maltster and brewer is the amount of nitrogenous material that is extractable from ground malt with warm water (say 65.5 °C). This is called Total Soluble Nitrogen. In the first day or two of germination, this value increases but, eventually, it reaches a peak and then declines because it is being elaborated into embryo protein. Another important parameter is the 'soluble nitrogen ratio' – that is the soluble nitrogen as a percentage of the total nitrogen of the corn. This indicates how much of the protein of the corn is extractable and how much remains in the spent grain. Thus if a maltster selects from one variety of barley a series of batches showing a spread of total protein or nitrogen, the soluble nitrogen ratio will tend to decrease as the total nitrogen increases. This demonstrates that the nitrogenous materials of high-protein barleys are used relatively wastefully in brewing, quite apart from their relatively low carbohydrate content.

There is a surprising array of proteases present in germinating barley. At least five are endopeptidases, enzymes able at any peptide linkage to cleave randomly the chain of amino acids making up the protein. Their activity increases about 20-fold during germination. Some of these endopeptidases have thiol groupings (i.e. —SH) at the active site of the molecule. They are inhibited by oxidative conditions, heavy metals and iodo-compounds (Table 3.2). Other endopeptidases are metallo-enzymes

Table 3.2. *Malt proteinases and peptidases*

		pH optimum	Important
Proteinase 1 (with thiol groups in active site)		3.9	Yes
Proteinase 2 (with thiol groups in active site)		5.5	Very
Proteinase 3 (with metallic coenzyme)		5.5	Yes
Proteinase 4 (with metallic coenzyme)		6.9	Not very
Proteinase 5 (with metallic coenzyme)		8.5	No
Carboxypeptidase 1	differ in the particular	5.2	Very
Carboxypeptidase 2	sequences of amino acids	5.6	Very
Carboxypeptidase 3	at the end of the protein	5.0	Very
Carboxypeptidase 4	chain that they will attack	4.8	Very
Neutral peptidase 1	differ in the particular	7.2	Not very
Neutral peptidase 2	sequences of amino acids	7.2	Not very
Neutral peptidase 3	at the end of the protein	7.2	Not very
Neutral peptidase 4	chain that they will attack	*c.* 7.0	Not very
Alkaline peptidase 1	differ in the particular sequences of amino acids	8.0–10.0	No
Alkaline peptidase 2	at the end of the protein chain that they will attack	8.8	No

whose activity can be seriously impaired by chelating the metal present in the molecule.

Also present in the germinating corn are peptidases which cleave amino acids or simple peptides from the proteins. The most important are the carboxypeptidases which liberate amino acids. They are so named because they attack the chain at the end where there is a free carboxyl group. Among the wide range of amino acids liberated is proline (which strictly speaking is an imino acid) (Fig. 3.6). This can only be utilised by yeast under aerobic conditions and therefore after a brewery fermentation, the beer is rich in proline compared with other amino acids.

Overall the situation is that if we start with barley with 100 parts by weight of nitrogenous material, the malt produced may well have 94 parts and the rootlets 6 parts. When the malt is extracted with water at

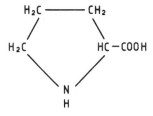

Fig. 3.6. Proline.

65.5 °C, some 40 parts solubilise and 54 parts remain in the spent
grains. Of the 40 parts, about 0.8 are represented by amino acids. Much
of this, apart from the 0.3 parts of proline, will be used for yeast
growth. Some of the more complex nitrogenous material will precipitate
as hot trub or hot break – or during subsequent cooling as cold trub or
cold break or as haze (turbidity) during beer production. Some, on the
other hand, will be present in the beer and play an important role in
foam formation when the beer is poured into the customer's glass.

Starch

Turning to the carbohydrates, the most important material is starch
(found in starch grains). In most instances where starch is enzymically
degraded in industrial situations, the starch has either to be gelatinised
by heat or subject to intense mechanical damage. Barley starch
gelatinises at 52–9 °C but, during germination processing, the
temperature is only around 15 °C. The starch-splitting enzymes – the
amylases – therefore act in malting without gelatinisation.

There are two forms of starch present in the grains, amylose and
amylopectin (Fig. 3.7). The former is a glucose polymer comprising
some 1000–4000 units of glucose; it therefore has a molecular weight of
about 200 000–800 000. Each glucose is linked to its neighbour by what
is termed an $\alpha 1,4$ bond. (Cellulose is a similar molecule except that the
bonding is $\beta 1,4$.) This linkage means that the reducing group of glucose
at the number 1 position is no longer effective. A molecule of amylose
has no more reducing power than a single molecule of glucose because
there is only one functional reducing group – at one end of the
molecule. At room temperature, the chain of glucose molecules takes
the form of a spiral and the coils are of such dimensions that an iodine
molecule fits neatly within them. When amylose is treated with iodine
dissolved in potassium iodide solution, the iodine finds a position in the
coils and the amylose–iodine complex has a blue–black colour. If the
complex is heated, the spiral from of the amylose is temporarily lost
and the iodine will not stain it.

Amylopectin is also a polymer of glucose but is bigger, with a
molecular weight in excess of 500 000. Most of the units of glucose are
linked by $\alpha 1,4$ bonds but there are occasional instances of another
bond, $\alpha 1,6$. The effect of this is to make the molecule branched but, like
amylose, there is only one functional reducing group in the molecule.
Iodine stains amylopectin but produces a reddish colour.

During malting, the barley starch is degraded, mainly to a mixture
of polyglucose molecules that are somewhat less complex than
the originals. The amount of simple sugars released for embryonic
respiration and biosynthesis is limited. Amylopectin tends to be

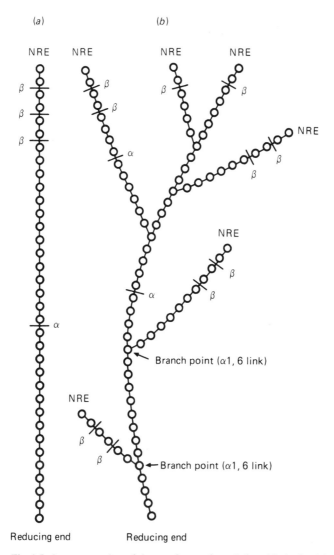

Fig. 3.7. A representation of the two forms of starch found in barley (*a*) straight-chained amylose and (*b*) branched amylopectin. Each circle represents a glucose unit and possible points of attack for α and β amylases are shown; NRE indicates a non-reducing end.

degraded preferentially compared with amylose. The enzymes able to degrade the non-gelatinised starch in barley appear to be (i) phosphorylase, (ii) α glucosidase, (iii) α amylase, (iv) β amylase and (v) debranching enzymes (Fig. 3.8). During the kilning of malt, the activities of these enzymes are drastically reduced, if not eliminated,

1. Phosphorylase (in embryo) – Inorganic phosphate needed, attacks α1-4 links → starch chain shortened at non-reducing ends by one unit plus glucose-1-phosphate
2. α glucosidase (in embryo) – Water needed for hydrolysis, attacks α1-4 or α 1-6 links → starch chain shortened by one unit at non-reducing ends plus glucose
3. β amylase (in embryo and aleurone) – Water needed for hydrolysis, attacks α1-4 links → starch chain shortened by two units at non-reducing ends plus β maltose
4. α amylase (in aleurone) – Water needed for hydrolysis, attacks α1-4 links → starch chains cleaved randomly to give mixture of dextrins plus a few sugars
5. Debranching enzyme (in aleurone) – Water needed for hydrolysis, attacks α1-4 links → debranching of amylopectin to give mixture of dextrins plus a few sugars

Fig. 3.8. The action of phosphorylase, α glucosidase, α amylase, β amylase and debranching enzymes on starch.

with the exception of α amylase and β amylase. The phosphorylase attacks the non-reducing ends of the starch molecules, not only cleaving a glucose molecule but also phosphorylating it to glucose-1-phosphate. This simple molecule is then available to the barley embryo. In the case of α glucosidase, the non-reducing ends of the starch molecules are again attacked to yield glucose. It is thought that glucosidase action makes it easier for α and β amylase to be effective on the raw starch. Debranching enzymes have the ability to cleave the α1-6 bonds and therefore have relevance to amylopectin.

The most important enzymes in malting and brewing are the α and β amylases (Table 3.3). They are so-called because they yield a carbohydrate product with a carbon 1 bearing its hydroxyl group in the α position or the β position respectively. But this difference is completely overshadowed by others. The α amylase is a metallo-enzyme and an endo-enzyme while the β amylase is a thiol-enzyme and an exo-enzyme. Even more important, the α amylase attacks randomly, hydrolysing any α1-4 linkage except (i) those close to a branching point and (ii) close to the end of the molecule. Thus, in the case of amylose, the enzyme yields straight-chained molecules of differing lengths. With amylopectin, the products are a mixture of branched and unbranched molecules. The effect of this cleavage is to lower the size of the original starch molecules very markedly; this reduces viscosity of the starch significantly. Each product has a functional reducing group and therefore the reducing ability of the degraded starch increases quickly.

In contrast, β amylase attacks the starch molecules at their non-reducing ends, cleaving β maltose, a disaccharide reducing sugar. This action is of course hindered by the α1-6 branch points of

Table 3.3. *Comparison of malt α and β amylases*

	α Amylase	β Amylase
1. Attack on starch chain	Randomly (except near chain ends and branch points); an endo-enzyme	Cuts off maltose from non-reducing ends of molecules; an exo-enzyme
2. Glucosidic link attacked	α1,4	α1,4
3. Products of attack	Mainly dextrins, few sugars	β maltose
4. Production of reducing groups	One per attack	One per attack
5. Production of non-reducing ends	One per attack	One per attack
6. General requirements	Calcium ions	Reducing conditions to maintain thiol groups
7. Inhibitors	Calcium sequestrants	Heavy metals and sodium iodoacetate
8. Optimum pH	5.5	5.2
9. Optimum temperature for most rapid actions	70	60
10. Presence before germination	Not present in mature barley grain, begins to form during germination	Present in mature barley grain but active enzyme increases during germination

amylopectin so that β amylase action leaves branched molecules. The main consequence of β amylase action however is to provide maltose sugar, a readily diffusible carbohydrate that can be used by the barley embryo. To the maltster, it is also important as sweetness in malt-extracts used for food. To the brewer, it is an easily fermented sugar, the main constituent of his wort.

The products of α amylase are mainly complex carbohydrates called dextrins, branched and unbranched. β amylase also yields branched dextrins, but more importantly maltose. It is not surprising that α amylase is often referred to as the dextrinogenic enzyme and β amylase the saccharinogenic enzyme. The two enzymes work in concert, the α amylase providing new non-reducing ends for the β amylase to attack. Nevertheless their action during malting is surprisingly limited. About 15–18% of the starch of the endosperm is solubilised during malting and of this some 11–12% diffuses to the embryo for respiration and biosyntheses. Only 4–6% is converted into simple sugars and dextrins. Nevertheless, the starch reserves are breached; the malt is an effective package of enzymes and readily degradable carbohydrate.

The β amylase is present in the barley before it germinates although much of it is in a bound, ineffective form. In contrast, the α amylase is synthesised once germination begins, triggered by the action of gibberellins. During the germination period, the proportion of α to β amylase steadily increases. Furthermore, at kilning, α amylase is more thermostable than β amylase. Strongly kilned malt can therefore be deficient in β amylase.

Endosperm cell walls

The cell walls of the starchy endosperm consist primarily of hemicelluloses which are insoluble in hot water, and gums that are soluble. It is possible that there is virtually a continuous spectrum of compounds rather than a clear-cut distinction. Cell wall materials make up about 10% of the weight of the barley corn and about a fifth of these materials are water-soluble. Looking at the walls from a chemical viewpoint, some molecules are polymers of pentoses (5 carbon sugars) and called pentosans (Fig. 3.9). Other molecules are polymers of glucose and some others may be mixed pentose and glucose (heteropolymers). The most important constituents to maltsters and brewers are the glucose polymers called β glucans. Indeed, barley

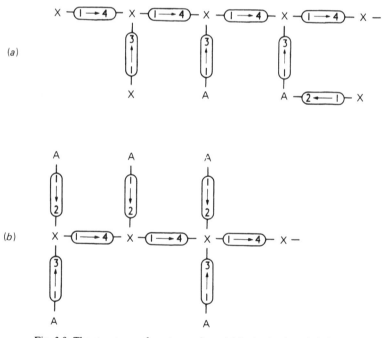

Fig. 3.9. The structures of pentosans from (*a*) barley husk and (*b*) barley endosperm. A: arabinose; X: xylose; each ellipse represents the linkage between the pentose sugars.

(a)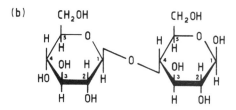

(b)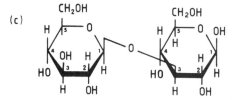

(c)

Fig. 3.10. The structure of β glucan from barley. (*a*) Part of the molecule; $\sim$ shows β 1–3 links and — indicates β1–4. (*b*) The formula for cellobiose (glucose β1–4 glucose). (*c*) Laminaribose (glucose β1–3 glucose).

varieties rich in these compounds may be rejected for malting. About $\frac{3}{4}$ of the linkages present in β glucans are β1-4 and the remainder mainly β1-3 (Fig. 3.10). They are gums that solubilise during the production of wort and may precipitate as a jelly during fermentation or post-fermentation steps. There are, however, several enzymes that are capable of degrading them; some are present in the raw barley (such as cellulase which attacks β1-4 links), others are initiated during germination (such as laminarinase, which attacks β1-3 links). They survive to some degree the process of malt kilning. The glucanases are endo-enzymes, such as cellulase and laminarinase, or exo-enzymes splitting off glucose. The important point is that the β glucans must be degraded to the point that the products are soluble in cold as well as hot water. They will not then precipitate in beer. Of course if any fermentable sugars are produced, that is a bonus.

Fats

Another group of compounds present in the endosperm is the lipids or fats. About 3.5% of the weight of the corn is lipid and approximately 10% of this is consumed in the respiration of the embryo. It is mainly deposited in the embryo and in the aleurone layer. Just over $\frac{2}{3}$ of the lipid is in the form of neutral fats (especially triacylglycerols), about $\frac{1}{4}$ as

(a)
$$CH_2O-CO-R_1$$
$$CHO-CO-R_2$$
$$CH_2O-CO-R_3$$

(b) $CH_3(CH_2)_{14} \cdot COOH$

(c) $CH_3(CH_2)_7 CH=CH (CH_2)_7 COOH$

(d) $CH_3(CH_2)_4 CH=CH CH_2 CH=CH (CH_2)_7 COOH$

(e)
$$CH_2O-CO-R_1$$
$$CHO-CO-R_2$$
$$CH_2O-PO_3H-(CH_2)_2 \overset{\oplus}{N}-(CH_3)_3$$
$$OH^{\ominus}$$

(f)

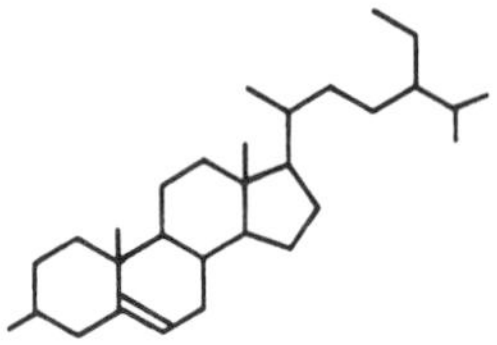

Fig. 3.11. Types of lipid present in barley and malt. (*a*) Generalised formula for a neutral fat (triacylglycerol with R_1, R_2, R_3 as fatty acids, as shown in (*b*), (*c*) and (*d*)); (*b*) palmitic acid, saturated fatty acid; (*c*) oleic acid, unsaturated fatty acid and (*d*) linoleic acid, doubly unsaturated; (*e*) lecithin, a phospholipid and (*f*) β-sitosterol, a sterol.

phospholipids and the rest as glycolipids (Fig. 3.11). Of particular interest to the brewers are the unsaturated fatty acids present in some of the neutral fats. These are important in yeast-membrane synthesis and in beer staling. The three groups of lipids are degraded by esterases, phosphatases and glycosylases respectively, while the fatty acids are oxidised by peroxidases and oxygenases.

Phosphates

Finally mention should be made of the phosphate-containing compounds in the corn which make up about 1% of the dry weight. They include phospholipids, nucleic acids and a curious compound

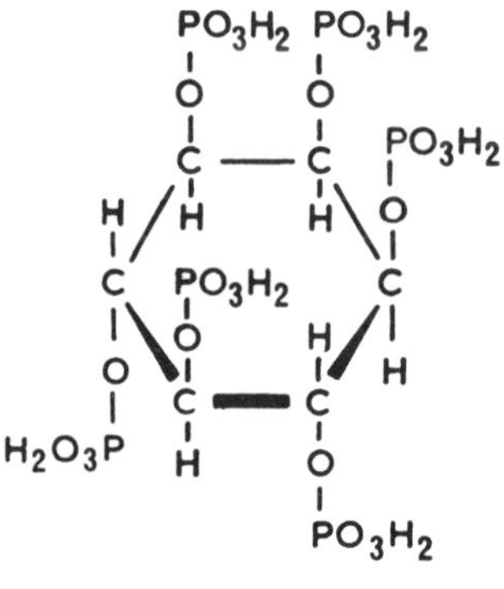

Fig. 3.12. Phytic acid.

called phytic acid. The last accounts for about half of the corn's phosphate and is a hexaphosphate of the sugar alcohol inositol (Fig. 3.12). It happens that inositol is a B group vitamin and many strains of yeast have a requirement for it. Phytic acid is degraded by phytase in the corn to yield myoinositol and phosphoric acid; the latter is used by the corn embryo but the brewer is more interested in it being used by yeast. Another point is that phytic acid has a very high affinity for calcium ions. As will be seen in the next chapter, the capture of calcium ions leads to a release of protons and hence the environment becomes more acidic.

Interactions

It must not be thought that degradation of protein, starch cell wall and fat are independent. Starch breakdown is aided by partial solubilisation of protein, mobilisation of fat and breakdown of the β glucans. In turn, β glucans appear to be attacked by a carboxypeptidase called β glucan solubilase. It severs the ester linkages between proteins and β glucans, at the same time as rendering high molecular weight β glucans soluble.

Kilning

The germination process is arrested by the maltster simply by drying out the malt corns. He may choose to have less well modified malt for lager malt, better modified for ale malt, with very well modified malt for distilling and vinegar manufacture. Another choice available to the maltster in his processing relates to the drying regime. Long, cool drying leads to a pale malt with much of its enzyme content intact whereas a rapid hot drying produces a dark malt deficient in enzymic activity.

The physics of drying are complex but they hinge on the fact that a sample of malt has a characteristic water vapour pressure at any particular temperature. The vapour pressure rises significantly with rising temperature. Thus a combination of high air flow and high temperature will dry quickest, a fact well known by anyone hanging out clothes to dry. It is usual to express the water vapour pressure of grain in terms of the relative humidity (RH) of the surrounding air (i.e. the RH of air in equilibrium with the moist grain at the prevailing temperature). Evaporation of water from the surface cools the grain and this latent heat of evaporation is 2.26 kJ g^{-1} at 100 °C. Because we want to preserve the enzyme activity of the grain, this cooling effect is important in hot drying air. Indeed, moist grains should never rise to temperatures above 38 °C. As the grain temperature rises, so does the rate of diffusion of moisture to the surface of the corns, because it is constantly being evaporated.

The factors that affect the rate of grain drying include (i) the volume of air passing through the bed of grain, (ii) the depth of the bed of grain, (iii) the weight of water to be removed from the bed of grain, (iv) the temperature of the drying air, (v) the relative humidity of the drying air and (vi) the hygroscopic character of the malt. Taking each point, a high rate of air flow is desirable but is relatively expensive; in the same way, a shallow bed is desirable but impractical. The quantity of moisture to be removed depends on specifications. Thus a tonne (dry weight) of malt with 45% moisture needing to be dried to 5% moisture will have to lose 400 kg of water. The temperature and moisture of the air are interrelated as already stated. Finally the hygroscopic character of the malt refers to the comparative difficulty of taking out the last few percentage of moisture from the hygroscopic materials such as gums and husk.

In particular, the maltster must never allow the air flowing through the grain bed to become saturated with water vapour. If he does, water will be condensed on the corns and will permeate downwards. In this connection, it must be remembered that the latent heat of evaporation will cool the air significantly. There will therefore be a big difference between the temperatures of the air entering the kiln ('air-on') and that leaving the kiln ('air-off'). The kilning starts with an air-on temperature of 50–60 °C which initially warms the kiln and bed of grain. Later, the lower layers of the bed begin drying and the barley becomes progressively drier from the bottom to the top of the bed of grain. At this free-drying stage, the water is being removed from the barley without restriction, and for economy's sake, the air flow is adjusted so

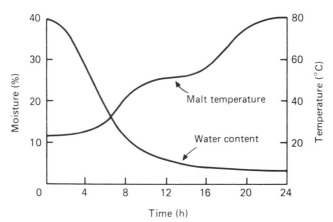

Fig. 3.13. Graph illustrating the loss of water from malt and its temperature during a typical one-floor kilning.

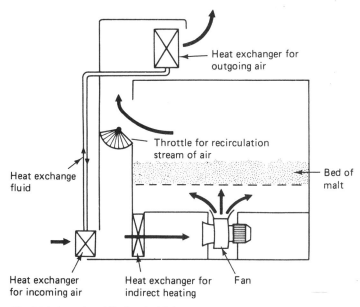

Fig. 3.14. A modern kiln fitted with heat exchangers and capability of indirect heating.

that the RH is 90–95% in the air-off. When about 60% of the water has been removed, (with malt at, say, 25% moisture) the bound nature of the residual water hampers further evaporation. At this 'break point' stage, the air-on temperature is increased and the air flow reduced (Fig. 3.13). The heat stability of the enzymes is now greater than it was with malt at 45% moisture. At the 12% moisture level, all the water remaining in the grain is bound so the air-on temperature is increased to 65–75 °C and the air flow is again reduced. The moisture uptake is slow and economy dictates that much of the air is recirculated (Fig. 3.14). Finally, at 5–8% moisture, depending on the barley variety, the air-on temperature is increased to 80–100 °C until the required colour and moisture content is achieved. Typically lager malts are dried to 4–5% moisture but ale malts to 2–3%.

Special coloured malts may be kilned using a totally different regime because the aim is to achieve colour and flavour. Enzymic activity is of no consequence. The malt is therefore either roasted or stewed and then roasted.

The selection of malt for brewing

Malt is the major raw material in brewing; it provides appropriate substrates and enzymes to yield a soluble extract or wort. The malt

Table 3.4. *Some typical specifications laid down by brewers for various malts; an indication of permitted variations is provided for ale malt*

	American 6-row malt	European 2-row malt for lager	European 2-row malt for ale
Moisture (%)	4.0	3.5	2.0 ± 0.2
Extract after fine grind (% on dry weight)	77.0	79.0	80.0 ± 0.4
Extract after coarse grind (% on dry weight)	75.3	77.4	78.6 ± 0.4
Total nitrogen (%)	2.1	1.75	1.70 ± 0.7
Soluble nitrogen (ratio to total nitrogen)	40.0	39.0	39.5 ± 1.0
Diastatic power (degrees Lintner)	140.0	75.0	65 ± 5
DU α-amylase (dextrinsing units)	40.0	35.0	–
Colour (degrees EBC)	3.8	2.9	6.0 ± 1.0

must provide extract cheaply and easily. It must also provide husk as an effective filter bed for clarifying the wort. The extract or wort composition determines the success of the yeast fermentation as well as contributing significantly to the flavour, colour and stability of the final beer.

In order to obtain raw materials that are as uniform as possible and are cost-effective, brewers set tight specifications. These specifications depend on analytical methods and therefore malt analysis has two functions, (i) to estimate the brewing value of a malt and (ii) to be the basis of commercial transactions. The main specifications are given in Table 3.4, along with typical values. From what has already been stated, it is not surprising that the brewer needs values for (i) moisture, (ii) total nitrogen or protein, (iii) extract from finely ground and coarsely ground malt, (iv) soluble nitrogen content of the extract, (v) enzyme activity, (vi) fermentability of the extract and (vii) colour. Some brewers also expect a measurement of hardness of the malt and of viscosity, β glucan content and amino acid content of the extract. It is thought by some authorities that extract values, the ratio of soluble nitrogen to total nitrogen of the malt and hardness of the malt are the parameters giving most information on malt quality.

Gibberellic acid

It will be recalled that gibberellins secreted by the barley embryo stimulates the aleurone layer to produce a new range of enzymes. A very similar plant hormone called gibberellic acid was discovered many years ago in Japan in connection with research on dwarf forms of

Table 3.5. *The advantages and disadvantages of adding gibberellic acid before or during germination* (*at 0.25 mg kg⁻¹ barley*)

May break dormancy
Increases the extract levels of the malt (by say 1–3%)
Reduces germination time (to 2–3 days)
Makes it possible to malt poorer (feed) barleys – especially with the abrasion technique
May increase malting loss (especially by greater respiration rate and greater rootlet growth)
Increases green malt volume
Increases modification (may get too high a level of soluble nitrogen)
Increases colour (disadvantageous for pale malts).

plants. Later it was shown that the hormone may be produced from a fungus, *Gibberella fujikuroi* (syn. *Fusarium moniliforme*).

The method of manufacture is as follows. A selected strain of the fungus is inoculated into an aqueous medium containing glucose 2% (w/v), the principal salts of which are ammonium chloride, magnesium sulphate and potassium dihydrogen phosphate. Batches of up to 25000 l are processed at 28–30 °C with perfusion of the medium with an oxygen, nitrogen and carbon dioxide gas mixture, usually about 0.5 volume of air per volume of culture per minute. The pH is initially at 3.5–4.5, falls to 3.0 during active growth of the fungus but rises again to at least 4.5 as the microorganism autolyses. Addition of further glucose may take place during the lengthy fermentation of 17–20 days. With autolysis, the gibberellic acid is released into the medium and is extracted with a ketone that is immiscible in water. Alternatively the acid is adsorbed onto a solid alkali–metal bicarbonate.

Although gibberellic acid has had a disappointing record in agriculture, it has been used successfully in malting. It might be expected to augment the natural gibberellins of barley; this it does, to enhance embryonic growth and metabolism. Even more importantly, it stimulates the aleurone layer to produce the hydrolytic enzymes in greater quantity. But the effects are indeed wider because gibberellic acid can also be used effectively to break dormancy and to speed up the entire process of germination. There are however, disadvantages in that the rootlets and acrospire grow more extensively, there is general over-modification, increased respiration and greater heat output (Table 3.5). Maltsters have found ways of minimising the unwanted effects and yet getting clear advantages. Thus the dose is restricted to the range 0.025–0.25 mg of gibberellic acid per kilogram of barley. It is added either to the final steep water or sprinkled over the steeped barley after it has been cast into the germination box. Some maltsters will also suppress the effects of gibberellic acid in increasing respiration and the output of proteolytic enzymes by using it in conjunction with sodium or potassium bromate. The dose is 100–500 mg kg^{-1} of barley. The potassium bromate is all reduced to bromide during the germination and kilning processes.

Malt and malt extracts outside brewing

Some 50000 tonnes of malt extract are produced each year in Britain. It is made by a milling and mashing process almost identical to that of a brewery but the wort recovered from the spent grains is concentrated to over 80% solids. Diastatic malt extracts are rich in malt enzymes or 'diastase'; they are dried in a single evaporator in a process that begins at 35 °C and rises to 45 °C. Such extracts are used in cereal syrup manufacture and, to a limited extent, in food manufacture such as confectionery. Non-diastatic extracts are used more extensively and are cheaper to produce because a three-stage evaporator with considerable energy economy is used. Temperatures of the extracts rise to 80–85 °C during drying and their enzymes are largely inactivated. These extracts are used for milky night-cap drinks, baking, biscuit manufacture, home-brewing, blancmange manufacture, and industrial enzyme manufacture. They are also employed as flavour carriers on a wide range of foodstuffs such as breakfast cereals.

4   Water – its functions in brewing

The water of brewing centres

Water makes up some 95% of the content of beer and therefore with a world-wide annual beer consumption of 850 Mhl, some 85 Mm³ of drinking water is drunk in the form of beer. Yet this very large volume (equivalent to a lake of 1 m depth and 9 km by 9 km area) gives no indication of the amount of water consumed by the brewing industry. Large volumes are sometimes stored (Fig. 4.1). Much is used for cleaning; considerable volumes are also employed in steam raising, evaporation, the loss of cooling and heating water to sewers, and the water left in spent materials (Fig. 4.2). Breweries vary much in their efficiency in using water. The most sparing are reported to use just less than four times the volume of beer produced, but many breweries use as much as ten times.

Water is becoming increasingly expensive (Table 4.1) and so is the treatment of waste water. There are therefore powerful financial incentives to economise in the use of water and the yield of effluent. Furthermore there are environmental reasons for such economies, for instance keeping natural water tables high, lowering emission of water vapour and reducing water pollution.

Brewing centres developed where the water available suited the kind of beer being produced. Thus the high gypsum (calcium sulphate) content of Burton-on-Trent was ideal for the full-flavoured strong pale ales first produced by the monastery brewery. In contrast, the rather soft water of Pilsen in Czechoslovakia was ideal for the production of pale lagers and indeed such lagers are commonly referred to as 'Pilsner' or 'Pils' wherever they are brewed in Europe. Water rich in calcium bicarbonate (temporary hardness) proved excellent for the production of darker, more mellow beers and therefore Munich, London and Dublin became renowned for such beverages.

The development of chemical analysis at the end of the nineteenth and early part of the twentieth century led to a knowledge of the ionic composition of natural waters (Table 4.2). At the same time, procedures for softening water were becoming available; salt mixtures that could also be added to softened water so that the waters of Burton-on-Trent or elsewhere could be mimicked. With an increasing knowledge of the

41

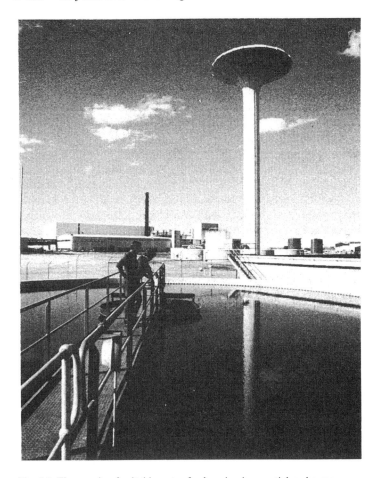

Fig. 4.1. The supply of suitable water for brewing is essential and some
breweries store large volumes as shown by the water tower in this photograph,
taken at Swan Brewery, Perth, W. Australia. Treatment of the brewery effluent
is another important feature and is shown in the foreground.

biochemistry of malting and wort production over the past 80 years, it
has become apparent that two ions are particularly important in the
control of pH. These are calcium and carbonate (or bicarbonate).
Calcium ions also have many other roles to play in brewing, as will be
mentioned later. Brewers therefore often adjust the chemical
composition of their brewing water. This helps them to control pH,
provide sufficient calcium ions and to adjust the concentration of other
ions important in beer flavour.

It has already been mentioned that cleaning and steam raising use
large volumes of water; the optimum chemical composition of this

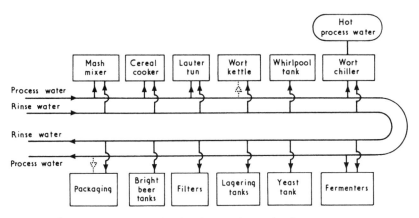

Fig. 4.2. Flow diagram showing the use of water in a brewery.

Table 4.1. *Cost (pence m⁻³) of water and effluent treatment by the Severn Trent Water Authority 1978–83*

	Water abstracted from private wells	Measured water from public supplies	Standard effluent charges[a]
1978/79	1.04	12.7	9.85
1980/81	1.48	17.6	12.22
1982/83	1.76	22.7	13.97

[a] COD and SS (notional strengths) for the standard effluent in 1978/79 were 403 and 342 respectively and were reduced progressively to 345 and 329 in 1982/83.

Table 4.2. *The ionic composition of water in brewing centres (mg l⁻¹)*

	Na^+	Mg^{2+}	Ca^{2+}	Cl^-	SO_4^{2-}	HCO_3^-
Burton-on-Trent	54	24	352	16	820	320
Pilsen	32	8	7	5	6	37
Munich	10	19	80	1	6	333
London	24	4	90	18	58	123
Dublin	12	4	119	19	54	319
Dortmund	69	23	260	106	283	549

water is very different from that of brewing water. A first consideration might suggest that the water should be completely free of salts. In practice, water free of salts tends to corrode metal pipes by solubilising undesirable amounts of the metal. It is therefore preferable to have water which is slightly hard and which will form a passive film on pipes. Such water can then readily be deionised cheaply for boiler-water feed, used as it is for cleaning and treated with appropriate salts for brewing.

Chemical and microbial contamination

It is estimated that half of the world's population (about 2 billion people) have no access to safe drinking water and about 80% of all disease is thought to be water-related. Despite the widespread incidence of malaria, river-blindness and bilharzia, much of the disease is a direct result of human activities. Thus typhoid and cholera may well become endemic in various parts of the world. Between 1980 and 1990, however, the United Nations Organization plans to spend $300 billion to provide safe drinking water and sanitation for the entire world population.

Not only microbial but also chemical contamination of water is widespread and therefore breweries must take particular care in selecting and treating the water that they use. Much of it is abstracted from wells, and is therefore derived from rain or melted snow that has penetrated not only soil but also the underlying rock. Wells are bored in rocks that hold water (aquifers). They are usually of a coarse, porous texture and are often ramified by fissures. The ionic composition of the water depends largely on the chemical content of the rocks through which it has permeated. Thus Permo-Trias rocks such as Keuper sandstone deposited during desert-like conditions have a high salt content. Porous sandstones may effect base-exchange and impart iron salts to the waters. In contrast, the water abstracted from limestones and chalks is rich in carbonates of calcium and magnesium.

Some breweries depend on rivers, lakes or even canals for their water supply and such water is more readily contaminated by organic materials and living organisms than is carefully maintained well water. Nevertheless both may be affected to some degree by the artificial fertilisers and chemical sprays used in agriculture and by chemical contamination from industrial operations in the catchment area. Of particular concern are (i) nitrates and nitrites derived from fertilisers, (ii) chlorinated hydrocarbons, detergents, mineral oil, arsenic, lead, mercury and chromium salts and other toxic materials from industrial operations and (iii) domestic sewage. Standards of purity have therefore been drawn up for potable water, first nationally and now internationally (Table 4.3). The concern about nitrites is that they will react with certain nitrogenous compounds, such as amines, to give carcinogenic compounds called nitrosamines. Nitrates, readily converted to nitrites by many bacteria found in both natural waters and in brewery worts, are of equal concern. Yet nitrates and substances

Table 4.3. *International standards for drinking water (1971) plus additional limits applied to European drinking water (1970) in mg l^{-1}* [a]

	Permissible	Excessive
Total solids	500	1500
Total hardness (as $CaCO_3$)	100	500
Fe^{3+}	0.1	1.0
Mn^{2+}	0.05	0.5
Cu^{2+}	0.05	1.5
Zn^{2+}	5.0	15.0
Ca^{2+}	75	200
Mg^{2+}	30–150[b]	150
SO_4^{2-}	200	400
Cl^-	200	600
F^-	0.6–1.7[c]	–
NO_3^-	–	45
As	–	0.05
Cd^{2+}	–	0.01
CN^-	–	0.05
Pb^{2+}	–	0.1
Hg^{2+} (total)	–	0.001
Se	–	0.01
Anionic detergents	0.2	1.0
Mineral oil	0.01	0.3
Phenolic substances (as phenol)	0.001	0.002
Polynuclear aromatic hydrocarbons (μg l)		0.2
Gross α emission	–	3 pCi l^{-1}
Gross β emission	–	30 pCi l^{-1}
pH	7.0–8.5	< 6.5 and > 9.2
Ba^{2+}	1	
Cr^{6+}	0.05	
H_2S	0.05	
NO_3^-	0.05	
NH_4^+	0.05	
Dissolved O_2	> 5	
Free CO_2	0	

[a] US standards are almost identical with those listed but there are some additional limits especially in connexion with chlorinated hydrocarbon.
[b] Depends on the SO_4^{2-} level, the 30 being applicable to 250 mg of SO_4^{2-} l^{-1}.
c Depends on maximum daily air temperature, highest values for 10–12 °C (50–3.6 °F).

giving rise to nitrates are often applied in excess in intensive farming. Industrial contamination of water is under stricter control but mistakes do occur and are not always immediately noticed.

With respect to water other than that from bore-holes, the population of living organisms is normally eliminated by filtration and chlorination. Bore-hole water is not necessarily so treated and therefore contamination with effluent, particularly domestic sewage, is serious. Therefore routine bacteriological analysis is usually practised. This concerns detection of more or less harmless bacteria that normally inhabit the intestines of humans and other animals. Such bacteria belong to the family Enterobacteriaceae and are so abundant in faeces (10^8–10^9 cells g^{-1}) that very small traces of faecal material can be demonstrated by bacteriological techniques. The numbers and viability of any pathogenic bacteria, such as typhoid- or cholera-producing organisms, are in comparison very much lower. Thus the rationale adopted is that if the non-pathogenic faecal bacteria are absent from water, it is reasonably certain that the pathogens are. The faecal coliform bacteria are usually characterised by growing on a lactose medium at 44 °C and producing gas, acids and the protein-decomposition product, indole. Some however fail to grow at 44 °C but do at 37 °C. It must be stressed that distinguishing and counting the various coliform bacteria is not easy and requires experience.

Softening and deionising

Temporary hardness can be reduced by boiling, especially if the boiling water is aerated (Eqns 4.1 and 4.2).

$$HCO_3^- \rightleftharpoons CO_2 + OH^- \tag{4.1}$$

$$Ca^{2+} + 2HCO_3^- \rightleftharpoons CO_2 + CaCO_3 + H_2O \tag{4.2}$$

This helps to drive off the carbon dioxide and precipitate calcium carbonate. The measure is less effective when magnesium ion is present because magnesium carbonate precipitates less well and is more soluble. Another traditional method is to add carefully controlled doses of slaked lime to the water so that the carbonate is precipitated (Eqn 4.3).

$$Ca^{2+} + OH^- + HCO_3^- \rightleftharpoons CaCO_3 + H_2O \tag{4.3}$$

A corresponding treatment for permanent hardness is to treat the water with soda ash (Eqn 4.4).

$$Na_2CO_3 + CaSO_4 \rightleftharpoons CaCO_3 + Na_2SO_4 \tag{4.4}$$

Acid treatment of water eliminates temporary hardness and is often employed (Eqn 4.5) by breweries.

$$HCO_3^- + H^+ \rightleftharpoons CO_2 + H_2O \tag{4.5}$$

Deionising is a process involving resins that are capable of either acid- or base-exchange. Zeolites, which are natural resins, have been largely superseded by synthetic resins such as polystyrenes. For the removal of temporary hardness, a weakly acidic (cationic) resin would be employed (Eqn 4.6).

$$RH_2 + Ca(HCO_3)_2 \rightleftharpoons RCa + 2H_2O + 2CO_2 \qquad (4.6)$$

The resin, when completely converted to the calcium and magnesium form, can be regenerated with acid treatment. With permanently hard water, an anionic resin would be used (Eqn 4.7)

$$RNa_2 + CaSO_4 \rightleftharpoons RCa + Na_2SO_4 \qquad (4.7)$$

and would be regenerated with caustic soda treatment. It is possible to remove both temporary and permanent hardness by using the cationic resin first, degassing the water to remove carbon dioxide and then treating it with the anionic resin. In recent years an alternative to deionising has been reverse osmosis using a cellulose acetate or nylon membrane that prevents larger ions from passing through it but permits water and smaller ions. Naturally, a considerable pressure is needed (say 30–60 bar) to drive water through the membrane.

The importance of calcium and bicarbonate ions

Temporary hardness in brewing water is normally reduced to less than 25 mg l^{-1} by either acid treatment or lime addition. This is because when wort is boiled the bicarbonate yields carbon dioxide by taking up hydrogen ions (Eqn 4.8).

$$CO_3^{2-} \underset{H^+}{\nearrow} HCO_3^- \underset{H^+}{\nearrow} H_2CO_3 \longrightarrow CO_2 + H_2O \qquad (4.8)$$

This uptake leads to a reduction in acidity and, therefore, the pH level rises.

Malt provides a considerable amount of phosphoric acid when inositol hexametaphosphate (phytin) is degraded by the enzyme phytase. Phosphoric acid readily ionises and Eqn 4.9 shows that hydrogen ions are released.

$$H_3PO_4 \underset{H^+}{\searrow} H_2PO_4^- \underset{H^+}{\searrow} HPO_4^{2-} \underset{H^+}{\searrow} PO_4^{3-} \qquad (4.9)$$

In the presence of calcium ions, the very insoluble calcium phosphate precipitates. This precipitation induces further molecules of phosphoric acid to dissociate and, at the same time, release hydrogen ions. Thus the solution becomes progressively more acidic and the pH of the wort falls.

Calcium ions are also important in stabilising malt α amylase, which, with malt β amylase, is the most important enzyme in the degradation of starch in mashing. Without calcium, the α amylase fails to operate normally. Because calcium ions precipitate phosphates and reduce wort pH, other enzymes that operate better at lower pH values, such as β amylase and some of the peptidases, will be more active in the presence of calcium. Also, polyphenols will be extracted to a lesser degree at lower pH so that derived beers are less astringent and less coloured. Yeast cells and trub flocculate more readily in the presence of calcium ions and, therefore, clarifying wort and beer is facilitated. Finally, in the presence of calcium ions, there is precipitation of calcium oxalate crystals, thus avoiding the uncontrolled release of dissolved carbon dioxide from beer (called gushing). Although magnesium ions have generally similar effects to calcium ions, their effectiveness in reducing pH is far less because magnesium phosphate is more soluble than calcium phosphate. Magnesium ions are, however, essential for the functioning of certain yeast enzymes. For instance magnesium is a cofactor for pyruvate decarboxylase, the enzyme which mediates in the production of acetaldehyde.

Cleaning and sanitising

During the brewing process, there are opportunities for inorganic salts and organic materials to precipitate and adhere to the surface of vessels, pipes and other equipment in contact with wort and beer. Principally, these deposits are salts of calcium and magnesium, denatured protein and yeast deposits. It is necessary to clean equipment in order to prevent a building-up of these deposits, especially on heat-transfer surfaces. Even more important is removal of this soil before it provides nutrients and protection for contaminating microorganisms. Strictly speaking, it is possible to sterilise this soil but that only makes its subsequent removal more difficult and, in any case, the sterilisation is only temporary.

The important rule is clean first and sanitise later. A typical cleaning sequence involves first a wash with water. The water does not have to be absolutely clean – it can be water that has been used in the final rinse. This is followed by spraying, at high velocity, a sanitising fluid held at 80–5 °C. For stainless steel equipment this fluid comprises 2% aqueous caustic soda, admixed with sodium hypochlorite which not only sterilises but also aids the cleaning. In order to dissolve calcium salts, sodium gluconate may be added; to keep insoluble particles of dirt in suspension and prevent their deposition, sodium tripolyphosphate may also be added. Usually the sanitising fluid or detergent is returned to a reservoir pending further use and is brought up to strength. The vessel is then sprayed with a cold, clean water rinse; this slightly soiled water is subsequently held in a reservoir tank before being used as first water rinse. In rigorous programmes of cleaning, the vessel or pipes are then sprayed with cold sterilant which might be an iodophor (an acidic iodine-yielding formulation), before being given a final cold water spray.

In the past 20–30 years, the cleaning of vessels has become automated. Labour is expensive and manual cleaning is not always reliable. Breweries have therefore moved towards enclosed vessels fitted with sprayballs and high pressure rotating jets. The programme of opening and closing valves, spraying rinse and sanitisers and returning solutions to reservoirs is selected. It is programmed into a microprocessor which sends signals at the appropriate times to activate valves and pumps of the 'Cleaning in Place' (CIP) system. This system results in considerable economy of water use compared with manual cleaning. The manual energy of cleaning is replaced by chemical energy, heat and by mechanical energy of high pressure sprays.

Steam is also used for sterilisation but can only be fully effective if it is saturated and operates in hot equipment. There must be ample opportunity for condensate to escape as the equipment heats up. At least 30 min steam treatment at 1 bar over pressure after the equipment has heated above 100 °C is necessary to achieve sterilisation of a cleaned piece of equipment. Steam is relatively expensive, particularly if used on a vessel in a cold room. It must be free of chemical contamination. Finally, its effects are nullified if the equipment is subsequently cooled with non-sterile water.

Water in cooling and heating

When the brewer wishes to cool clarified hopped wort, he normally uses a plate heat exchanger with cold water running counter-current to the hot wort. As a result, a great deal of hot water (at say 70–85 °C) is produced. This is used either as mashing-in and sparge water or is employed to heat such water. It is also used for cleaning purposes. Further supplies of hot water may also be produced by passing cold water through a heat exchanger in the wort kettle flue-pipe heated by the steam driven from the wort during wort boiling.

Most breweries use dry saturated steam (at about 150 °C and 3.5 bar over pressure) for heating but some employ high pressure hot water (in the range 145–170 °C at about 17 bar over pressure). Steam installations are cheaper but are complicated in that the rate of steam use is determined by the rate at which the steam can be condensed. There is only restricted opportunity for building up a reservoir of energy and, therefore, steam-generating plant has to be flexible in its response to demands for heat energy. High pressure hot water systems circulate to and from the heater in a closed loop. The volume of water in the system represents a huge reservoir of energy so that sudden demands can easily be met. There is also less problem in controlling energy input into the brewing equipment, there is no condensate to drain and solids tend not to bake onto stainless steel surfaces to the same extent as with steam heating.

Effluent treatment by breweries

Breweries often may treat their own effluent to meet the standards needed for discharging it, after treatment, into open waterways. Alternatively they may choose to discharge effluent to the public authority sewage works without any treatment. There is, too, the possibility of partial treatment by the brewery.

Effluent strength is measured by (i) the concentration of suspended solids (SS) and (ii) the concentration of materials that can be oxidised chemically by boiling with potassium dichromate and concentrated sulphuric acid (chemical oxygen demand or COD). The reason for measuring COD is that when effluent enters a waterway, dissolved oxygen is consumed by aerobic microorganisms as they metabolise the organic material. Thus the more organic material is present, (in other words where there is a high COD), the more dissolved oxygen is used. High levels of organic material may completely deoxygenate the water and would lead to the death of aerobic organisms. It is therefore necessary to restrict COD levels of effluents discharged into natural waterways to, say, 10–20 mg l^{-1}. Restriction of suspended solids is also required because not only do they usually represent organic material but they may settle in natural waterways to give an anaerobic sludge. Typically, bulked brewery effluents have an SS value of 240 mg l^{-1} and a COD value of about 1800 mg l^{-1}. Brewery effluents are usually in the pH range 3.5–5.5 except for discharges of spent caustic-based sanitisers whose pH values may be as high as 10.

The cost of discharging effluent to the sewers is calculated by the local authority on a formula which takes into account (i) the volume of effluent, (ii) the cost of transporting effluent to the sewage works, (iii) the suspended solids concentration, (iv) the cost of removing these solids, (v) the COD level and (vi) the cost of reducing COD levels to approved final levels. There may be restrictions on the pH and temperature of the effluent and penalties if SS and COD exceed certain limits. It is therefore important for the brewery to maintain volume, SS and COD values to a minimum. This can be achieved by restricting the discharge of spent materials such as malt particles, hop fragments, excess yeast, trub and the lees (sediment at the base of a vessel) from beer tanks. It is also important not to discharge weak worts or spoiled beer. As far as possible, spent materials should be collected in spent

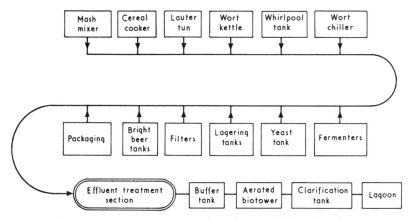

Fig. 4.3. Flow diagram showing the production of effluent in a brewery.

grains and sent to farms for animal feed. Weak worts and spoiled beer can be incorporated into pig swill or recycled appropriately in the brewing process.

If a brewery decides to treat its own effluent, it is desirable to filter it roughly and to bulk the outfalls (Fig. 4.3). This necessitates a buffer tank but the dwell-time should be only a few hours otherwise microbial digestion with attendant unpleasant smells will develop. The effluent may then be either treated aerobically, which is relatively common, or anaerobically which is rare but of increasing interest.

The aerobic digestion depends on a large population of microorganisms which is able to take up both soluble and colloidal organic materials from the effluent and metabolise them to mainly carbon dioxide and water. The energy derived from the metabolism enables the microbial cells to grow. There are two basic types of process available of which the most venerable is the percolating filter system. This comprises a 2 m bed of stones contained within a circular wall which is naturally ventilated. The effluent is sprayed from rotating distributor arms above the bed and trickles between the stones which are coated with a slimy population of microorganisms (Fig. 4.4). Although the dwell-time may be only 30 s, there can be substantial reduction in SS and COD. However, the percolating filter operates poorly in the conditions of variable flow, variable composition and fluctuating pH of effluent, quite apart from the high SS and COD values. A modern counterpart is a tower which is very loosely filled with sheets of rigid plastic material on which the microorganisms grow. The effluent trickles down the tower counter-current to rising air.

More common is the activated sludge system which depends on a high concentration of microorganisms that flocculate. These sludge

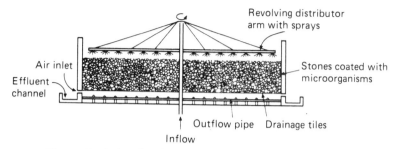

Fig. 4.4. Vertical section through a percolating filter.

organisms are kept in suspension by compressed air or mechanical agitation. High rates of oxygen transfer can be maintained to aid aerobic metabolism of the effluent (Fig. 4.5). In the process, the sludge organisms grow prolifically and the population has to be kept roughly constant by removing some of it. The sludge is difficult to dewater and is not popular as a fertiliser because, among other drawbacks, it tends to smell and often has a high metal content. The sludge system is expensive in its use of energy for aeration (more than 50% of a brewery's electricity may be used for this purpose). Additionally a

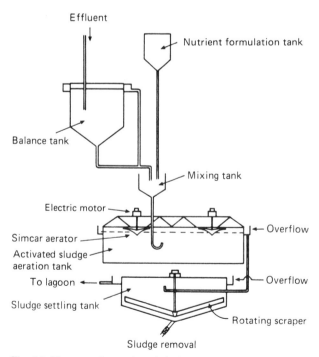

Fig. 4.5. Diagram of an activated sludge plant.

settlement device for removing SS has to be installed downstream from the activated sludge plant.

A further method is to use an anaerobic system of digestion within an enclosed container. The bacteria used for the digestion tend to be of two general types: one type producing acetic, propionic and other fatty acids from the metabolism of the effluent organic material; the other type yielding methane and carbon dioxide. Growth is slow and the yield is about 0.55 g l^{-1} but the COD values are reduced by about 75% and the SS by 50%. Furthermore the process yields a gas which can be used in a gas engine, boiler or heat exchanger. The disadvantages of the process is the long time it takes to start up and its sensitivity to variations in loading and effluent composition.

The capital cost of a brewery treatment plant is high, for instance the anaerobic digestion equipment for a brewery of 1 Mhl beer production per year would be in the order of £0.5 M. Furthermore all these processes, whether anaerobic or aerobic, yield water which will require further treatment before it is suitable for discharge into waterways. It is not surprising therefore that many breweries rely entirely on local authority sewage works for the treatment of their effluent.

5   Sweet wort production

Grain reception

Most large breweries receive their malt and solid adjuncts in bulk
deliveries by road or rail vehicles. They maintain something like 3 days'
to 3 weeks' stock. The raw materials are usually elevated before being
weighed, screened, passed through magnetic separators and weighed
again (Fig. 5.1). In this way the material is cleared of dust, foreign
objects and anything metallic (which might cause sparks when it strikes
equipment).

The raw material is held in silos or storage bins, usually of steel or
concrete, with smooth side and conical bases. Within the silos, the raw
material is kept at a constant temperature (say 10–15 °C) and at a low
moisture level. This discourages the development of insect colonies.
Malt moisture levels are in the range 2–5% while those of wheat flour,
maize flakes and maize grits are 10–12%. Insects such as certain weevils
and grain beetles are able to develop even under these conditions and
their metabolism yields water, carbon dioxide and heat. The water and
heat promote faster development. Warning of their presence is therefore
sought by means of sensitive temperature probes within the silo.
Movement of the raw material through the screening equipment tends
to even out temperature but does not eliminate infection. Chemical
disinfection of empty silos and grain-handling equipment may be
necessary on occasions.

Another hazard in grain handling is the dust which is formed. This
has to be aspirated by air cyclones and trapped in appropriate filters.
Cereal dust can cause serious damage to the mucous membranes of
workers. It is also dangerous because of the risk of explosions. In the
region of grain handling, mechanical and electrical equipment must not
generate sparks.

Milling

The object of milling is to crush malt to produce grist. (ground or
milled grain, a gritty flour). It is important that the husk is kept as
entire as possible but the endosperm is ground to particles that readily
release their extract. If the husk is badly distintegrated, it is less

54

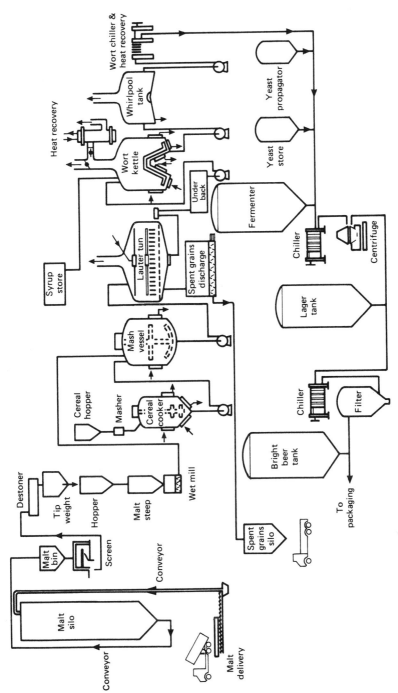

Fig. 5.1. Flow diagram of a brewery showing grain reception, wort production, fermentation and post-fermentation equipment.

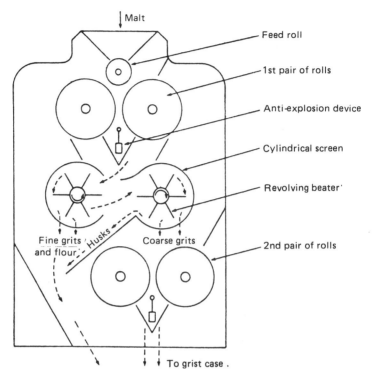

Fig. 5.2. A 4-roll mill with screens.

effective in forming a permeable filter bed during wort recovery from the mash. Also, the broken husk easily releases more tanning material than is desirable. Turning to the endosperm fragments, it is necessary to have grits that readily hydrate and release their enzymes and other cell contents so that degradation can take place rapidly. Very small particles would be ideal from this standpoint but tend to pack together to provide an impermeable bed so that wort runs off slowly and incompletely. The fineness of grinding therefore depends on the type of wort-recovery equipment being used; one with a deep bed requiring, in general, coarser particles than one employing a very shallow bed.

Both dry and wet mills are common in breweries. The dry mills are of two principal kinds but both are roller mills. With well modified malt, the simpler roller mill comprising two pairs of contra-rotating rolls may well suffice (Fig. 5.2). Less well modified malt is often characterised by having hard ends and such malt needs a 6-roll mill that is able to detach the hard ends from the husk (Fig. 5.3). Large breweries often select 6-roll mills for their greater flexibility, even though malt with hard ends would never be entertained.

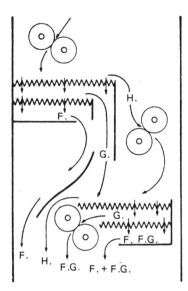

Fig. 5.3. A 6-roll mill with screens. H, husks; G, grits; CG, coarse grits; FG, fine grits; F, flour.

Roller mills provide endosperm particles differing in size from coarse grits at say 0.3–0.6 mm diameter to fine grits (0.15–0.3 mm) to flour (less than 0.15 mm diameter). The gaps between the rolls can be adjusted to keep the proportion of coarse grits low or alternatively the proportion of flour low. In general, the proportions of coarse:fine:flour range from 27:35:38 to 24:35:41.

Some breweries spray the malt with water or subject it to steam just before it enters the mill. The treatment makes the husk more pliable and therefore less prone to damage. A more extreme approach is to wet mill where the malt is steeped in water to raise its moisture content to 28–30% before the crushing rolls tear open the corns. Steeping should not occupy more than 30 min, and is usually only 5–10 min. The product of a wet mill is a slurry of husks and endosperm particles which is pumped or dropped into a mash mixer. This contrasts with dry milling where the dry product may be stored for several hours in a grist case before it is hydrated in the mashing processes. Some dry cereal adjuncts such as maize flakes and wheat flour pellets go through the dry mill along with the malt. Others such as maize grits are milled separately, normally in a simple 2-or 4-roll mill.

In traditional breweries, mills were mounted high in the building so that they were positioned above the grist cases and mashing equipment. Nowadays, the mill may be mounted at ground level and the grist emerging from it is conveyed mechanically or pneumatically.

Infusion mashing

The traditional mashing equipment for the production of ales is the
mash tun. Grist is fed from the grist case into what is called a Steel's
masher (Fig. 5.4). This is a hydrator comprising a large-bore tube about
46 cm diameter with a right-angle bend. The grist is sprayed with hot
water [2.7 hl $(100 \text{ kg})^{-1}$] in the first and vertical part of the tube and is
mixed with a revolving screw in the horizontal portion. Thus the
hydrated grist or mash falls into the mash tun like thick, somewhat
aerated porridge. The temperature of the mash at this stage is critical
because changing it without serious dilution with water is very difficult.
It has been established that the best mash temperature for this system
of mashing is in the range 62–7 °C, and usually is 65 °C. To achieve this,
the water used is some 4–5 °C higher.

Before the mash falls into the tun, the vessel is heated and partly
filled with hot water to a level just over the filter plates. The mash,
because it has entrained air, tends to float, an important feature of
traditional mash tuns. As the particles of endosperm hydrate, the
enzymes renew their attack on the partly degraded, and therefore highly
vulnerable, food reserves of the malt. In particular, α and β amylase
operate in concert to degrade amylose and amylopectin to produce
fermentable sugars and non-fermentable dextrins (Table 5.1). Reference
to Table 3.3 reveals that α amylase is more thermostable than β
amylase so that higher temperatures (say 67 °C) favour α amylase but
not β amylase. Similarly a pH level of 5.7 is more conducive to β
amylase and one of 5.3 would be more favourable to α amylase. In
practice, a compromise obtains so that both enzymes are effective. But

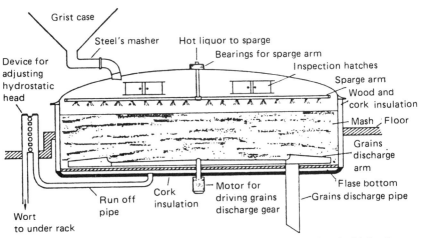

Fig. 5.4. Vertical section through an infusion mash tun equipped with Steel's
masher.

Table 5.1. *Production of soluble carbohydrates* [g $(100 \ ml)^{-1}$] *during mashing by* α *and* β *amylases*

Minutes	Fermentable sugars	Non-fermentable dextrins
0	1.1	3.5
25	4.0	2.8
50	6.9	4.3
100	10.8	3.7
150	11.2	4.0

Table 5.2. *Influence of mash temperature, concentration and water pH on the fermentability of sweet wort*

Mash temperature (°C)	60		65.6		68.3	
Mash thickness [g $(100 \ ml)^{-1}$]	67	39	67	39	67	39
Fermentable sugars (% of total solids)	73.3	76.1	67.4	71.2	64.4	65.0
Non-fermentable dextrins (% of total solids)	17.5	15.5	24.2	21.2	27.6	26.2
Mash water pH		4.0		4.5		5.5
Fermentable sugars [g $(100 \ ml)^{-1}$]		8.9		8.3		8.4

Table 5.3. *Optimum temperatures and pH values for infusion mashing*

	Temperature (°C)	pH
Greatest extract	65–68	5.2–5.4
Most fermentable wort	65	5.3–5.4
α amylase activity	70	5.3–5.7
β amylase activity	60–65	4.6 (mash)
Greatest yield of soluble nitrogenous materials	50–55	5.0 (wort)

brewers have control on the fermentability of the wort they produce by providing optimum conditions for β amylase if they wish to increase fermentability (Table 5.2). What is noteworthy is that the brewer is using the enzymes at the top of their temperature range. The enzymes are being denatured by the high temperatures but nevertheless are operating at or near their maximum rate. Therefore, over a short time span (say 30–120 min), they are at their optimum temperature. With respect to pH, the brewer can adjust this by the methods outlined in Chapter 4, usually by eliminating carbonate and bicarbonate ions in the brewing water and ensuring that there are adequate calcium ions present (Table 5.3).

In addition to amylase activity, there is also proteinase action. This is optimal at about 50 °C but, because the malt used is well modified, considerable protein degradation has occurred during malting. Nevertheless there is in mashing an important supplementation to this breakdown, even at 65 °C. This particularly applies to those proteinases that are exo-enzymes and cleave amino acids from the protein chains. They also operate better at pH values around 5.3 than at 5.7 and in thick mashes where they are more protected by substrate than in thin mashes. Thus the brewer has some measure of control. To enhance proteolysis, he would use lower mash temperatures, comparatively low pH levels, thick mashes and longer mashing times. In practice, it is necessary to compromise where the system of mashing selected demands higher temperatures or thin mashes or high pH levels.

In the mash tun it is possible to use flaked cereal or cereal flour as adjuncts at levels of 10% (or below) of the grist. The important considerations are that the starch present in the adjunct is in a state that can be degraded by malt amylase. Furthermore there must be sufficient amylase available to hydrolyse the starch quickly and effectively. For reasons given later, there is no wish on the part of the brewer to degrade adjunct protein providing that the starch is attacked.

Turning to the malt endosperm cell walls, there is restricted opportunity for further degradation at 65 °C. Some of the pentosan and β glucan material of the walls is soluble but much of it is not. The β glucan, as it is progressively attacked during malting and mashing, produces first of all smaller polymers soluble in hot water or hot wort, and later cold-water-soluble polymers. It is an embarrassment to the brewer to have the material soluble in hot wort but not cold wort. Not only does it increase the wort viscosity which makes wort recovery from the spent mash more difficult, this material comes out of solution as a viscous jelly at any time from wort cooling to the dispensing of the beer. It is therefore important to the brewer to either restrict β glucanase activity to the minimum or make sure that its action is complete in yielding molecules soluble in cold wort or beer. If β glucan is a serious problem, the brewer may have to add to the mash glucanase derived from commercial strains of bacteria or moulds.

Enzyme attack in the mash tun leads to progressive solubilisation of the contents of the grist particles, leaving only a small amount of undegradable material. The mash water around the particles not only dissolves the extractable material but also drains through the bed and is filtered by the husks. In consequence, the water above and below the plates becomes rich in soluble carbohydrate and nitrogenous materials. It has become sweet wort and can be drained from the mash tun, normally at a specific gravity of between 1.060 and 1.100. However, in order to keep the mash bed floating and to get satisfactorily complete extraction, it is necessary to spray, or sparge, the bed. Water of 68–72 °C is used and the rate of sparging more or less compensates for the rate of wort run-off from the tun. Thus the worts withdrawn become progressively weaker and when they reach, for example, 1.005 the brewer will cease sparging rather than take still weaker worts.

In order to keep the mash floating, the extraction of worts must not impose a strong hydrostatic suction. The mash tun's wort-withdrawal pipes are therefore provided with an inverted U tube and syphon breaker. The mash tun is also supplied with spent-grains-removal gear. A powerful electric motor drives a propellor-shaped plough which, in turn, pushes the spent grains through discharge holes in the filter plate assembly. Usually the grains are conveyed in larger diameter pipes by compressed air to a bin from which farmers' trucks can load the spent grains (p. 71).

Decoction mashing

The mash tun system, often called infusion mashing, is simple insofar as only one vessel is used and the mash temperature is held virtually constant. It is complex in that many biochemical and chemical engineering unit operations take place in the one vessel. Other systems of mashing involve separate vessels for mashing and wort recovery.

Traditional German brewing was required to cope with poorly modified malt. Although most malt used now is satisfactorily modified, the system devised has only been altered in detail. This is because gross departures would possibly lead to unacceptable changes in the

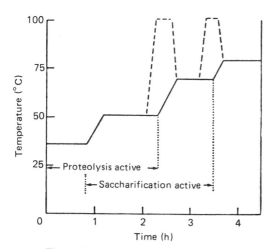

Fig. 5.5 Temperature changes during a double-decoction mashing procedure.

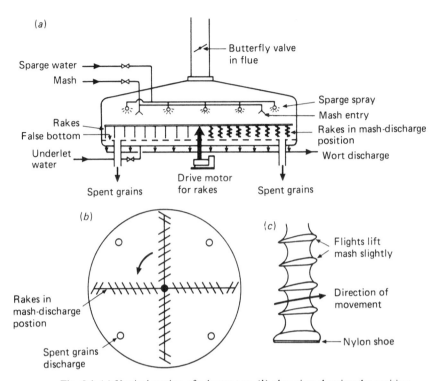

Fig. 5.6. (*a*) Vertical section of a lauter tun, (*b*) plan view showing the position of rakes for grains removal and (*c*) detail of a rake.

character of the worts and beers produced. The principle of the decoction mashing commonly used in Germany is to mash in the grist at a rather low temperature, say 40 °C, and then withdraw a quarter of the mash to a kettle and boil it. By mixing the boiling mash to the remainder of the mash, a step-wise increase in temperature occurs, possibly to 54 °C. This decoction procedure can be repeated, leading to an overall temperature of 65 °C. A final decoction would give a mash temperature of about 73 °C (Fig. 5.5). These temperatures provide for optimum conditions of proteolysis between 40 °C and 54 °C, optimum conditions for starch hydrolysis between 54 °C and 65 °C and finally, at 73 °C, optimum conditions for separating wort. There has been a tendency to reduce decoctions to one or two by a higher initial mashing temperature and use of third volumes in the mash kettle. This is a measured response to well modified malts.

The wort is separated from the spent mash in a vessel called a lauter tun (Fig. 5.6) or in a mash filter (Fig. 5.7). Lauter tuns are superficially like mash tuns but usually operate with only 0.5 m depth of mash (in contrast to the mash tun's 1.5–2.0 m depth of mash). The mash has to be thin [3.3–5.0 hl (100 kg)$^{-1}$] because it has to be pumped. Due to its

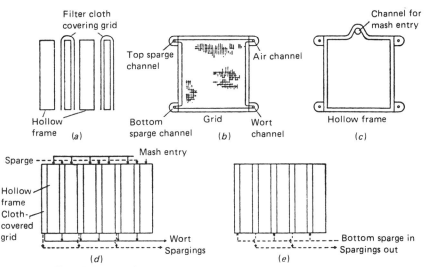

Fig. 5.7. Details of a mash filter. (a) Diagram of vertical section, (b) elevation of a grid or plate, (c) elevation of a frame, (d) early operations in the use of the filter, (e) later stages.

thinness, and the effects of pumping and boiling, decoction mash has no entrained air and therefore does not float. It sinks onto the lauter tun and plates; wort can only be induced to drain by frequent raking. The rakes are mounted from a vertical concentric shaft and are powered by an electric motor. They may be swung from their cutting position to one at 90°, in order to double up for spent-grains removal. Sparging is, in some instances, continuous but often is delivered at periods when the rakes are temporarily resting.

Mash filters take up less room than a lauter tun and are able to cope with finer ground malt. In recent years mash filters have been restored to popularity by exploiting automated mechanisms for separating and closing the heavy cast iron frames and plates plus the use of easily cleaned polypropylene filter sheets. A comparison between mash tuns, lauter tuns and mash filters is given in Table 5.4.

Table 5.4. *Comparison of infusion mash tun, lauter tun and mash filter*

	Mash tun	Lauter tun	Mash filter
General characteristics	Mash conversion and wort recovery in one vessel	Purely for wort recovery	Purely for wort recovery
Turn round time (h)	4–6	3	1.5–2.5
Coarseness of grist	Rather coarse	Moderate	Fine
Space occupied	Moderate	Large	Small
Mechanical simplicity	Very simple	Moderate	Complex
Brightness of worts	Good	Moderate	Poor

Double mashing

American malts tend to be well modified and high in enzymes and other nitrogenous materials. Consequently the brewers usually employ high levels of cereal adjunct to exploit the enzymes and dilute the unwelcome high levels of nitrogenous compounds. Such adjuncts are usually maize grits or rice grits, both of which require cooking to make their starch grains fully vulnerable to amylases. The American system (called the double mash system) therefore involves cereal cookers in which the grits are mixed with a little malt. The temperature is brought to 65 °C where the malt enzymes reduce the viscosity of the starch paste before the mixture is boiled. During this processing, the main malt mash is started at, say, 45 °C and this encourages proteolysis and some starch breakdown. When the contents of the cereal cooker are added to the main mash, the temperature rises to about 67 °C (Fig. 5.8). This is conducive to rapid breakdown of both malt and adjunct starch. The mash is then heated to 72 °C to reduce viscosity and pumped into lauter tun or mash filter where the wort is separated.

Temperature programming

Most breweries in the world use the double mash system, but some terminate it by raising the temperature from 67 °C to 72 °C with a single decoction. There are some however that use what is called temperature programming, including many of the larger British breweries. The grist is mixed with water in a mash mixing vessel at an

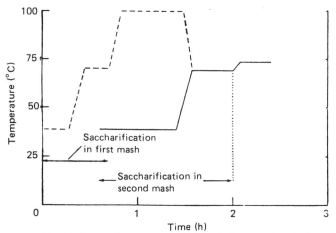

Fig. 5.8. Graph of temperature changes during a typical double mash procedure. The dashed line indicates the cereal cooker and the continuous line the malt mash vessel.

Table 5.5. *Comparison on infusion, decoction, double mash and temperature programming procedures*

	Infusion	Decoction	Double mash	Temperature programming
Materials normally mashed	All malt (well modified)	All malt (less well modified)	All malt in one mash (very well modified)	All malt (poorly modified)
Use of adjuncts	Usually 10% of maximum	Usually none but otherwise 10% of maximum	30–50%	30–50% if malt well modified
Boiling of malt mash	No	Yes	No	No
Proteolytic hold in region 40–50 °C	No	Yes	No	Yes
Number of vessels usually needed	1	3–4	3	2–3
Maximum number of brews per day in one set of vessels	5	8	12–14	12–14

initial temperature in the range 45–55 deg C. Heating jackets, coils or elements at the base and sides of the vessel are used to raise the temperature of the thin mash according to a predetermined programme, either linearly or in steps. Thus proteolysis and starch breakdown are accommodated before the mash is transferred to lauter tun or mash filter, at about 72 °C. A comparison of infusion, decoction, double mashing and temperature-programmed mashing is given in Table 5.5. The essential differences focus on the mash materials employed and on the time–temperature relationships employed to achieve the type of wort required by the brewer. In all cases, the fundamental biochemistry is the same.

Solid cereal adjuncts

Adjuncts are used by brewers for several reasons. They are often cheaper sources of extract than malt, but malt enzymes must be present in the mash in sufficient amounts to degrade the adjuncts. Where nitrogenous materials are supplied by the malt in excess, the use of adjuncts (which are almost always low in nitrogenous compounds) will dilute the levels in the final wort. Excess high molecular weight nitrogenous materials may lead to a beer which is prone to producing a haze when packaged. Amino acid levels in excess of the yeast's requirements in fermentation give increased opportunity for infection of the beer by lactic acid bacteria. Thus quantitative knowledge of amino acid requirements is essential for good brewing.

Many adjuncts will, when brewed with malt, give beers that are less satiating in taste and more refreshing. This is particularly important in the case of the more delicate lagers. There may also be improved flavour stability of the packaged beer, therefore prolonging the shelf life. Still another consideration is colour; most adjuncts reduce the final beer colour but some mentioned below are added particularly to increase colour.

The most commonly used adjuncts are the grits of maize and rice (Table 5.6). Maize or rice corns are washed, softened in steam and then abraded to remove the husk, embryo and aleurone layer. The remainder, the endosperm, is milled to produce grits of the appropriate particle size. Grits are rich in starch and contain far less fat and protein than the whole grain. Sorghum grits are also used as adjuncts to a limited extent. As has been mentioned, grits are cooked in a cereal cooker, normally with some malt but an industrial enzyme (bacterial α amylase) will substitute for reducing the viscosity of the starch slurry.

Flaked cereals are produced from grits by heating with microwaves, passing the hot grits through flaking rolls and then cooling. The heating means that the starch grains have been gelatinised and therefore are vulnerable to amylase attack without boiling. They can therefore be used in infusion and temperature-programmed mashing procedures.

Whole grains of cereals are also used as adjuncts. Thus, roasted barley is used in stout production. It produces extract and a great deal of colour due to melanoidin formation from carbohydrates and nitrogenous materials during roasting. Micronised (extremely finely ground) barley and wheat corns are also used in infusion mashing. The micronising gelatinises the starch and also produces colour and nutty flavours. Similar changes occur when whole grains are heated (torrified). Such adjuncts are inexpensive, provide a reasonable yield of extract and additionally the desired colour and flavours for certain beers. Wheat and barley flours are used in some infusion-mashing systems. They may be in the form of pellets. The flour is mixed carefully with the malt before and after the milling. Advantages in its use include inexpensive extract and improved beer foam because of the high glycoprotein content. The starch grains are physically and chemically affected by the rigorous milling and open to amylase attack.

The adjuncts described above require intake and storage facilities and sometimes special mills. It is not usually easy for a brewery to change from one type of adjunct to another; there must therefore be assurance of continuing supplies of good quality material. The mash-tun adjuncts

Table 5.6. *Characteristics of solid adjuncts used in mashing*

	Method of use	Moisture (%)	Extract (% dry weight)	Protein (% dry weight)	Lipid (% dry weight)	Gelatinisation temperature range (°C)
Maize grits	Need cooking	12	90	9.5	0.9	62–74
Rice grits	Need cooking	12	92	7.5	0.6	61–78
Refined maize starch	May or may not be cooked	11	103	0.5	0.05	62–74
Wheat flour	May or may not be cooked	11	86	8.5	0.76	58–64
Torrified barley	No cooking needed	6	72	14.5	1.6	–
Flaked maize (corn flakes)	No cooking needed	9	83	9.5	0.9	–

Table 5.7. *Composition of liquid adjuncts used in wort production (as a per cent of dry material)*

	Extract	Glucose	Fructose	Sucrose	Maltose + maltotriose	Unfermentable sugars
Solid sucrose	102	0	0	100	0	0
Invert sugar (Glucose + Fructose)	84	50	50	0	0	0
Maize (corn) syrup – high glucose	82	43	0	0	37	20
Maize (corn) syrup – high maltose	82	3	0	0	72	25

require just as much effort on the part of the brewer as malt but another group of adjuncts, the kettle adjuncts, offer considerable economies in the this respect (Table 5.7).

Liquid adjuncts

Maize and, to a lesser extent, wheat has been processed for many years to produce what are called 'glucose syrups'. To the chemist it is a misnomer because glucose is the name of a particular monosaccharide hexose sugar. A sugar technologist would refer to this sugar as dextrose (because it deflects to the right polarised light passing through a solution of the sugar). He uses the word 'glucose' for the products of starch hydrolysis and to him 'glucose syrup' means starch hydrolysate. Older methods of treatment involved acid hydrolysis of starch flour derived from maize grits. Present methods employ industrial enzymes. A starch slurry is liquefied by adding bacterial α amylase derived from *Bacillus subtilis* and heating to 85 °C (Fig. 5.9). The amylose and amylopectin are converted in an array of degradation products from glucose to dextrins. Further conversion is possible by cooling the syrup and providing the appropriate temperature and pH for the second enzyme that the sugar technologist selects. If the enzyme is malt amylase, then a pH of 5.0 and a temperature of 55–60 °C would be used. The result would be a maltose-rich syrup. On the other hand if the fungal enzyme amyloglucosidase is selected, using a pH of 4.5 and a temperature of 50–55 °C, the resulting syrup will be almost entirely glucose. An alternative to malt enzyme is the β amylase of *Bacillus polymyxa* and a suitable substitute for the mould debrancher is the enzyme pullulanase from the bacterium *Klebsiella aerogenes*.

Starch technology has provided yet another syrup recently, important in food but not in brewing. This is a fructose-rich syrup which is sweeter than sucrose. It is made from the glucose-rich syrup described above. After purification, the syrup is passed through columns packed with an immobilised enzyme called ketol isomerase; this converts just over 40% of the glucose into fructose. There are three fascinating aspects to the process. The first is that the immobilised enzyme is prepared from a bacterium that is killed by heat-treatment, yet the enzyme (which is intracellular) retains its activity. It remains attached to the cells so the column is packed with dead cells bearing an active enzyme. The function of the enzyme in the living cell is to convert one pentose to another by isomerisation. It so happens that the specificity of the enzyme is wide and, fortuitously, includes the isomerisation of glucose to fructose, although whether this conversion is carried out by the enzyme in the living cell is open to speculation. The final curious feature is that, in the USA, this starch-based product offers competition

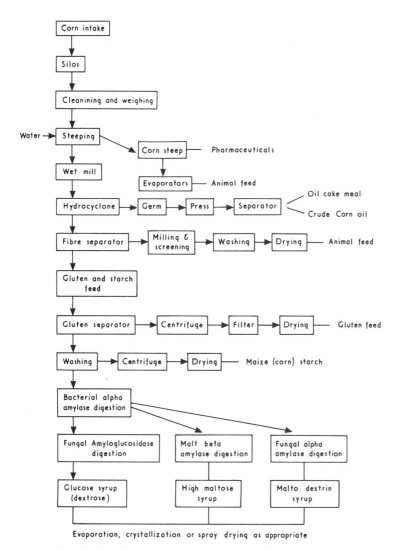

Fig. 5.9. Flow diagram of corn (maize) processing to yield various syrups.

to beet or cane sugar as a sweetener yet in the EEC its application is severely restricted by legislation.

In the brewery, the starch-based syrups are also in competition with those derived from cane and beet sugar. The latter are either virtually pure sucrose or acid-hydrolysed sucrose which is a mixture of glucose and fructose. The acid-'inverted' sucrose tends to crystallise from a syrup of 83% w/w solids and therefore must be stored at 40–50 °C. Incidentally, inversion refers to the change in the deflection of polarised light when the dextrorotatory sucrose is hydrolysed. Although the product glucose (syn. dextrose) is dextrorotatory like sucrose, the other product of the reaction (fructose) is strongly laevorotatory. Therefore during hydrolysis, the beam's rotation moves progressively to the left.

Syrups are usually stored at about 50 °C to lower their viscosity and therefore make pumping easier. They are used as adjuncts to the wort kettle or to the post-fermentation process. Because the extraction has been carried out by the syrup manufacturers, the brewer has merely to mix the material with his wort. In this respect, syrups are wort extenders. They can also be used to increase the gravity of the wort in the kettle, permitting what is called high-gravity brewing (described below).

The syrups vary in their fermentability, thus the starch-based ones are usually less than 100% fermentable whereas the sugar-based ones are normally fully fermentable. However there are strains of brewing yeast that give fermentation difficulties if the wort has a high proportion of glucose. The glucose itself is fermented completely by the yeasts but fermentation of the maltose and maltotriose afterwards is unsatisfactory. For this reason, some brewers prefer to use maltose-rich syrups instead of glucose-rich ones.

When sucrose, invert sugar or glucose is heated in closed digestor with a catalyst (usually an ammonium salt), caramel is produced. It is a mixture of burnt sugar and melanoidins. Some brewers use caramel for darkening their worts in the kettle or later in processing their beers, as an alternative to using roasted barley or roasted malts in the mashing process. Dyes are not employed for colouring beers but some are permitted in the UK for darkening ciders or soft drinks.

High-gravity brewing

There is considerable potential saving to the brewer if he produces wort of higher gravity than is necessary, ferments it and at the end of the brewing process dilutes it with water to normal strength. Thus heating a tonne of wort by 50 °C will use virtually the same energy if the specific gravity is 1.030, 1.050 or 1.070. Similarly cooling the wort by say 85 °C will use virtually the same refrigerant load whatever, within reason, the wort specific gravity is. Furthermore to produce say 1 Mhl of beer of OG 1.040, the brewer could produce 0.5 Mhl of wort of SG 1.080 and add water later, thereby using half the size of wort-production vessels and fermenters.

Two methods of high-gravity brewing are practised. The first is to use syrups to boost the specific gravity in the wort kettle. This demands additional heated syrup storage tanks, pumps and mains. The second method is to divert all worts of specific gravity below 1.010 collected from mash tun, lauter tun or mash filter to a special vessel. These weak worts are used in mashing in the next brew instead of water. A combination of diverting weaker worts and exploiting them for mashing gives a considerable boost to wort specific gravities.

There are difficulties. Any losses of worts and beers due to poor drainage or to spent materials holding wort or beer is more serious with high-gravity operation. Hop bitter substances are less well utilised in worts of higher gravity. Yeasts may produce beers of different flavour and aroma when fermenting high-gravity worts. Finally, it is not easy to blend water and beer on a continuous basis to achieve exactly the correct mix.

Spent grains

In most countries, spent grains must be dried before they can be used as animal feed. Otherwise the grains become mouldy. The drying is very expensive in its demands on energy. Although drying is practised in distilleries, no brewery in the UK dries spent grains. It is true that some animal feed specialists buy the brewery spent grains and dry them before compounding them with other animal feedstuffs. But most UK breweries sell their spent grains direct to farmers. The grains are also used by the breweries as a filter for effluent slurries containing spent hops, trub, yeast and tank bottoms. Thus the nitrogenous content of the grains may be enhanced by this further discharge of unwanted materials by the brewer and effluent costs reduced.

From 100 units of weight of malt, about 60 units of wet spent grains would be produced. If dried, the weight of grains would be about 15 units. As a food for cattle, 5 units of wet spent grains is equivalent to 1 unit of barley. The protein, fat and hemicelluloses are readily broken down by the microbes present in the gut of cattle. Table 5.8 shows the composition of feed value of fresh brewers grains.

Table 5.8. *Composition of fresh brewers' grains and their digestibility by sheep*

	Mean	Range
Dry matter (%)	26.3	24.4–30.0
Crude protein (% of dry weight)	23.4	18.4–26.2
Digestible protein (% of dry weight)	18.5	13.9–21.3
Crude fibre (% of dry weight)	17.6	15.5–20.4
Digestible fibre (% of dry weight)	7.9	6.6–10.2
Total ash (% of dry weight)	4.1	3.6–4.5
Lipid (% of dry weight)	7.7	6.1–9.9
Starch (% of dry weight)	11.6	–

Spent grains have been exploited for human breakfast food but alas the venture did not have lengthy success. The most amusing suggestion is that spent grains should be compressed into boards for the construction of edible hen houses. Another possibility is that industrial enzymes may be used to degrade the remaining carbohydrate of spent grains to yield simple hexoses and pentoses. On this, food yeast such as *Candida utilis* might grow to produce biomass.

6 Hops and wort boiling

Hop growing

Hops belong to the Cannabinaceae but, despite the relationship with *Cannabis*, the commercial hop *Humulus lupulus* contains no hallucinogenic substances. Female flowers develop on separate plants from the male flowers and, in most commercial hop-growing enterprises, male plants are eradicated. This gives rise to a situation where most commercial hops are unseeded. Nevertheless in Britain the majority of hop gardens have 1 male hop plant to every 200 female plants; this leads to almost complete seed-bearing (in commercial terms seedless means less than 2% seed by weight).

The hop plant is restricted to temperate climates and over-winters as a rootstock; it has long roots penetrating the soil which, in commerce, has to be deep and rich. In the spring, the plant begins to sprout from its crown. The shoots are adapted to climb any supports available and are referred to as bines. They have backwardly directed hooked hairs on their stems and petioles and they coil clockwise. The hop grower provides support for the bines by erecting strong timber posts (some 5–7 m high) to which are attached horizontal wires, usually at the top, roughly at the middle and at the bottom of the posts. These posts and wires run parallel with the rows of hop plants. Close to each rootstock, a hook is firmly anchored into the ground and to it is attached a number of strings (which are renewed each spring). These run to the wirework in such a way that the hops can twine to the top of the supports and yet there is ample room for a tractor to get between the rows of hops. Usually there are three strings from each hook and on each the grower encourages two bines to twine. The bines grow quickly from late April until July (in the northern hemisphere) to reach the top of the supports.

Rapid and heavy growth makes considerable demands on the soil, requiring annual additions of fertiliser equivalent to 90–100 kg of nitrogen, 10–16 kg of phosphorus, 60–80 kg potassium and 80–90 kg of calcium per hectare. Additionally the grower has to mulch the soil, spray the plants and drench the soil to restrict the development of various fungi, viruses, insects and acarines. The complex spraying of fungicides and insecticides is however restricted in order to ensure that,

73

Table 6.1. *Principal hop-producing countries and their yield in tonnes in 1982*

Federal Republic of Germany	42 500
USA	35 600
Czechoslovakia	12 800
UK	10 300
USSR	10 000
Yugoslavia	5 900
China	4 500
World total	145 000

Derived from information provided by Lupofresh Ltd, Wimbledon, UK.

when harvested, the female cones of flowers are free of spray residues. This in turn makes certain that the hop material used by the brewers is free of toxic materials. Table 6.1 lists the principal hop-growing countries.

Hop diseases

The most important diseases of hops arise from fungal infections of *Verticillium* wilt, downy mildew and powdery mildew. *Verticillium albo-atrum* is sufficiently serious that an outbreak at a hop garden may, because of Orders of Parliament, be isolated with respect to commerce and traffic. The infected plants will be burned. However, some areas are now suffering from endemic infection and have to plant only wilt-resistant strains. Conidial spores or mycelium of the fungus in the soil grow and enter the roots of the hop and ramify the vascular system of the entire plant. Leaves develop a characteristic tiger stripe and later detach. The base of the bine may thicken and then wither.

Downy mildew is caused by a fungus, related to that causing potato blight, called *Pseudoperonospora humuli*. Its ravages of hops in the original hop-growing area of the USA caused hop culture to be moved thousands of miles, from the eastern side of the continent to the western. At its worst it kills the rootstock while a late and mild infection may cause dark patches on the hop cones so that they have little market value. Powdery mildew (or hop mould) is, in contrast to the downy mildew, a disease associated with hot dry weather. The organism, *Sphaerotheca humuli*, produces conidial spores that germinate on leaves and cones to give characteristic greyish mycelia on the surface; later red spots develop from which erupt over-wintering spores.

Hop selection

Female cones develop from July onwards and are ripe for harvesting in September (in the northern hemisphere). The structure of the cone is shown in Fig. 6.1. It comprises a central stalk or strig which at each node bears four simple female flowers (bracteoles) and a sterile bract. Each bracteole has the capacity of developing a single dark-coloured seed, if pollination and fertilisation occur. But the commercial value of the cones resides in the tiny, almost microscopic golden glands scattered over the base of the bracteoles. These lupulin glands are rich in bitter resins and essential oils. The principal bitter resins are humulones or α acids.

Hops of commerce belong to four main groups: The Central European, Western European, the North American and the hybrids. Examples of them are Hallertau, Fuggles, Yakima Cluster, and Northern Brewer respectively. There are differences between hop varieties in growth form, growth vigour, yield of cones, yield of α acids, yield and composition of essential oils, and resistance to various diseases. Table 6.2 gives details of the characteristics of several modern varieties developed at Wye College, Kent which are hybrids of Western European and North American stocks. In general the purchasers of hops are interested in those varieties that are (i) particularly rich in α acids, or (ii) of attractive aroma or (iii) acceptable in both these respects. They are referred to as α-rich or kettle hops, aroma hops and mixed-function hops respectively. It will be appreciated that it is much easier to monitor for α acid content (which is readily measured) than for attractive aroma which is largely subjective assessment. Hop breeding is very different from that of barley breeding for many reasons. Because there are separate male and female plants, the characteristics of the female form of the male which provides the pollen must be known. Again, the rootstock rarely gives typical yield in its first and second year of growth. It is difficult, if not impossible to shift rootstocks from northern to southern hemisphere to get two crops each year. Finally, it must be noted that a rootstock once established is expected by the commercial grower to have a useful life of 5–15 years.

Hop picking and drying

Hops used to be picked by hand. The UK has its main areas of hop growing in Southeast England and in the West Midlands. These are conveniently close to the London and Birmingham conurbations and, until 1950, most hops were hand-picked by urban families enjoying (or suffering) a paid holiday in the country. Since then, machine picking has almost completely taken over (Fig. 6.2). The bines and strings are

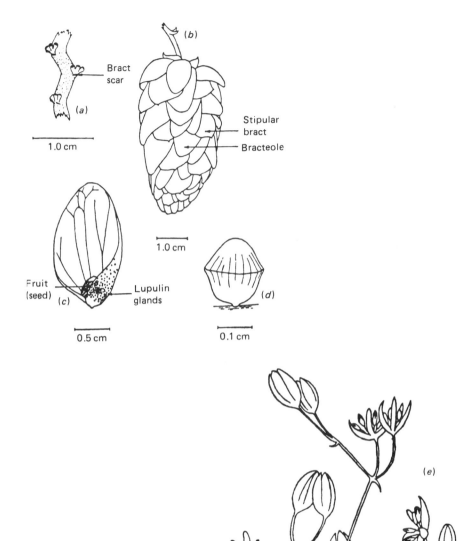

Fig. 6.1. Details of the hop inflorescence. (*a*) Part of the strig or axis of the female cone, (*b*) single mature hop cone, (*c*) bracteole with seed and lupulin glands, (*d*) lupulin gland and (*e*) male hop flowers.

Table 6.2. *Characteristics of some modern Wye College hybrid hops grown in UK (1981 values)*

	Resistance to diseases			Typical α acid (%)	Yield (kg α acid ha^{-1})
	Wilt	Downy mildew	Powdery mildew		
Target	Resistant	Susceptible	Resistant	11.5	200
Northdown	Susceptible	Some resistance	Susceptible	8.3, 11.2[a]	151, 182[a]
Challenger	Susceptible	Very resistant	Susceptible	7.7, 9.8[a]	150, 152[a]
Yeoman	Resistant	Some resistance	Susceptible	11.0	190[b]
Zenith	Susceptible	Some resistance	Susceptible	9.0	190[b]

[a] Seedless.
[b] Rough estimate.

cut at ground level and from the wire work, and laid in a tractor-drawn cart. They are carried to the picking shed where each bine is clamped onto a monorail. This carries the bine upwards so that it hangs vertically. It then carries it horizontally to the picker which flails the hops from the bine, along with leaves. Other equipment (by means

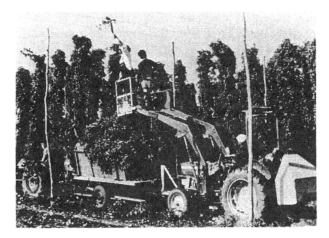

Fig. 6.2. Hop picking in Herefordshire, UK. The hop bines are cut at their base and from the supporting wirework at the top before being placed in the cart that carries them to the machine that detaches the cones.

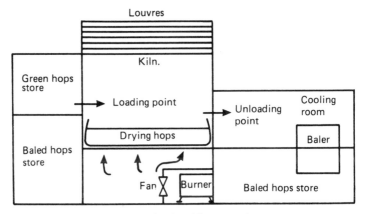

Fig. 6.3. Vertical section through a hop kiln or oast house.

of crude sieves and blasts of compressed air) separates cones from the lighter leaves.

The cones are then taken to the oast house or kiln where they are dried (Fig. 6.3). A typical drying regime would be 10 h at 60–65 °C. During this period, the air flow is maintained at a high level by the natural flue effect of the traditional hop kiln (oast house) or by an air fan. Drying the hop evenly is difficult because the strig retains its moisture tenaciously while the bracts and bracteoles tend to over-dry. In practice, the hops are dried to about 7% average and then permitted to pick up a further 1% moisture from the air so that the bracts and bracteoles become less brittle and less likely to detach. The strigs, being covered with bracts and bracteoles, take up little.

Hops are either baled or put into the traditional hop sacks or pockets carrying a stated weight (usually 79–87 kg). They are held in warehouses and are graded on the basis of appearance, aroma and α acid content. It is important to make the α acid determination as early as possible because the level falls due to oxidation. The bittering potential however drops much more slowly.

Hop chemistry

The composition of commercial hops is given in Table 6.3 and, of the components listed, the important materials for the brewer are the resins and the essential oils. Nevertheless tannins, proteins, amino acids and sugars are extracted during brewing, albeit in very small amounts. The resins present in fresh hops are mainly soluble in light petroleum (hexane) and these so-called soft resins principally comprise α acids and β acids. As hops age and oxidise, the proportion of petroleum-insoluble

Table 6.3. *Composition of commercial hops*

Water	10.0
Total resins	15.0
Essential oil	0.5
Tannins	4.0
Monosaccharides	2.0
Pectin	2.0
Amino acids	0.1
Proteins (N × 6.25)	15.0
Lipids and wax	3.0
Ash	8.0
Cellulose, lignin, etc.	40.4
Total	100.0

resins (called hard resins) increases, mainly due to chemical changes to the α and β acids.

The α acids, or humulones, are a family of compounds shown in Fig. 6.4. They differ in the side chain at carbon 2 in the six-membered ring. It is the α acids which are the most important source of bitterness in beer. The β acids or lupulones are a similar family of compounds but are less important. During the boiling of hops or hop products in wort, the α acids are chemically rearranged or isomerised as shown in Fig. 6.4. The compounds produced, iso α acids or isohumulones, are far more bitter and much more soluble than the α acids. In contrast the β

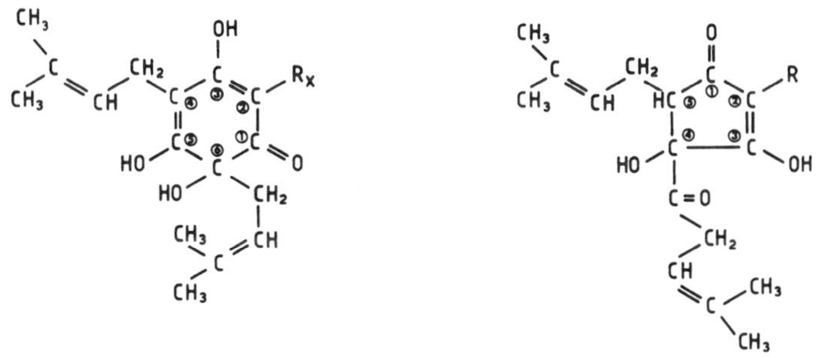

definition of R_x		name of $\underline{\alpha}$ acid	name of iso$\underline{\alpha}$ acid
$-CO \cdot CH_2 \cdot CH(CH_3)_2$	(isovaleryl)	humulone	isohumulone
$-CO \cdot CH(CH_3)_2$	(isobutyryl)	cohumulone	isocohumulone
$-CO \cdot CH(CH_3) \cdot CH_2 \cdot CH_3$	(2-methylbutyryl)	adhumulone	isoadhumulone
$-CO \cdot CH_2 \cdot CH_3$	(propionyl)	posthumulone	isoposthumulone
$-CO \cdot CH_2 \cdot CH_2 \cdot CH(CH_3)_2$	(4-methylpentanoyl)	prehumulone	isoprehumulone

Fig. 6.4. Structure of α acids and isoα acids.

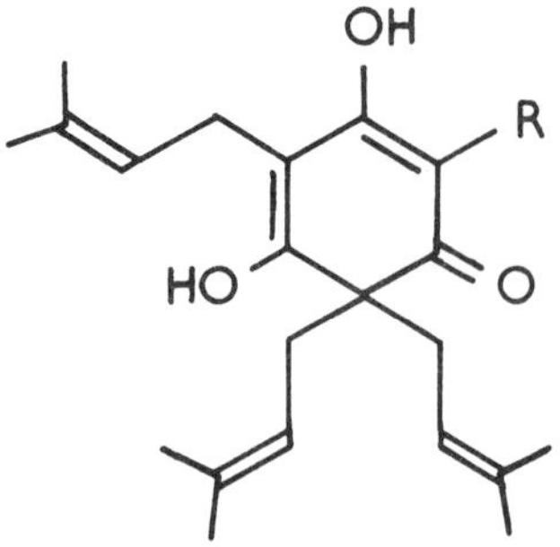

Fig. 6.5. Structure of β acids.

acids tend to oxidise during boiling to give an array of bitter and non-bitter derivatives (fig. 6.5). When hops age during storage, both α and β acids give rise to oxidised derivatives, some of which are bitter and others not. There is a tendency for the original structure to change with respect to (i) oxidation of sidechains, (ii) loss of sidechains and (iii) the six-membered ring contracting to a five-membered ring.

Essential oil of hops is a complex mixture of several hundred components; those soluble in hexane are terpene hydrocarbons (Fig. 6.6). The rest, soluble in ether, are compounds containing oxygen such as esters, aldehydes, ketones, acids and alcohols. Some are extremely potent, thus methyl thiohexanoate has a flavour threshold of 0.3 ppb. The essential oils have influence on both the flavour and aroma of beer although most of the oil added to boiling wort is lost by steam distillation. This is fortunate as a high level of essential oil would make beer undrinkable. Whether the oil enhances or detracts from the overall quality of the beer depends on the proportions of the many components. Essential oils oxidise during storage and become less attractive; furthermore they may speed up the oxidation of resins.

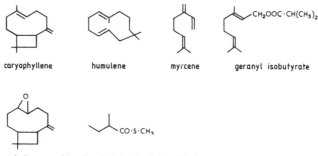

caryophyllene   humulene   myrcene   geranyl isobutyrate

carophyllene epoxide   S methyl. 2 methylbutanethioate

Fig. 6.6. Structure of typical essential oils of hops.

Hop products

Although many brewers use hop cones in their dried but otherwise
natural state, many hops are processed into pellets and extracts. The
pelleting process is simple in principle. In involves breaking up hop
bales and blending hop varieties as the brewer requests, hammer milling
the hops and then pelleting them in a die (Fig. 6.7). The pellets emerge
as dark green sticks (about 20 mm long and 10 mm in diameter) and
are vacuum-packed or packed in an inert atmosphere. Some are packed
into drums, others in large plastic or metallic foil sachets. The
advantage of pellets is that they store well in that the hops hardly
deteriorate through oxidation even at ambient temperature. They are
ready-blended and are easily weighed and conveyed.

For many years it has been possible to purchase hop extracts. The

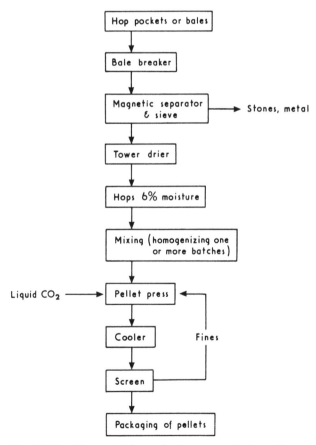

Fig. 6.7. Flow diagram of the production process for hop pellets.

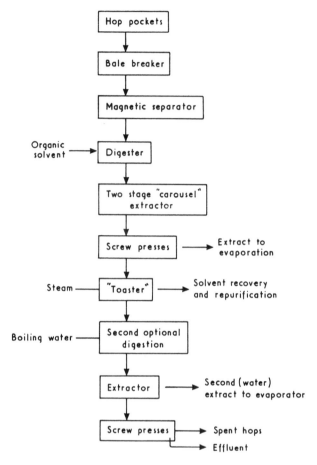

Fig. 6.8. Flow diagram of the production process for hop extracts using organic solvents.

extractant has been an organic solvent such as methylene chloride or ethanol. Although the solvent is recovered (Fig. 6.8), a very small quantity, possibly only a few parts per million, is left in the extract. Particularly in the USA there is concern about any chlorinated hydrocarbon being associated with a material to be added to a beverage or food. The organic solvent extracts both resins and essential oils. Some processes involve a second extraction with water so that tannins and pectins of the hops are also solubilised. In all cases these extracts tend to be dark green and viscous and have to be heated to make them flow and dissolve. However there are preparations where the extracts are made into a powder by mixing them with a suitable adsorbent such as silica gel or bentonite.

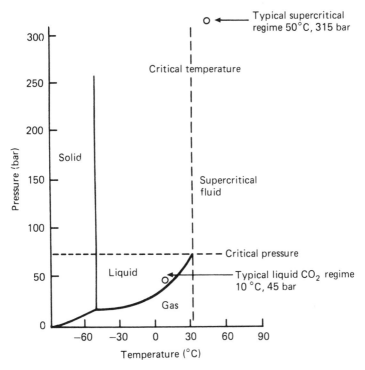

Fig. 6.9. Phase diagram for carbon dioxide showing the pressure and temperature characteristics of liquid carbon dioxide and supercritical carbon dioxide extractions.

In recent years, liquid carbon dioxide has been used as an extractant for foods such as coffee, tea, herbs, spices and fruit juices. It has even been used to remove from dried fish and meat various unpleasant impurities that cause off-flavours during storage. In the past 8 years, two processes have been described for the extraction of hops. To appreciate the differences between them, Fig. 6.9 shows the equilibrium properties of carbon dioxide. One process, called the supercritical, uses a temperature of 50 °C and pressure of nearly 400 bar. The liquid, or subcritical, carbon dioxide process in contrast operates at about 7 °C and a pressure of about 40 bar. Above 31 °C and 74 bar, carbon dioxide is no longer a simple liquid. With hops, the liquid carbon dioxide process tends to be selective so that no hard resins and tannins are extracted. Furthermore less water, fats and waxes are extracted than is the case in the supercritical process (Table 6.4). Hop α acids have a maximum solubility at $+7$ °C but extraction is poor from cone hops. Pelletised hops are therefore extracted after remilling. There are liquid carbon dioxide plants operating in Australia and Britain producing hop

Table 6.4. *Comparison of extracts prepared by treating hops with either carbon dioxide or organic solvents*[a]

	Supercritical extraction (CO_2)	Liquid CO_2 extraction	Organic solvent extraction
Total resins	77–98	80–98	15–60
α acids	27–41	35–55	8–45
β acids	43–53	25–35	8–20
Essential oils	1–5	3–10	0–5
Hard resins	5–11	0	2–10
Tannins	0.1–5	0–2	0.5–5.0
Water	1–7	0–2	1–15
Fats & waxes	4–13	0–8	1–20

[a] Components expressed as % w/w.

extract. At least one supercritical plant is manufacturing extract in the Federal Republic of Germany.

The first material to emerge from the column of hop powder is essential oil (Fig. 6.10); β acid begins to elute before all the essential oil has been recovered. Similarly, α acid emerges before the final essential oil has come off and before the β acid has been totally recovered. It is therefore possible to recover a fraction rich in essential oil, a fraction containing little oil but rich in both α and β acids and finally a fraction which is mainly α acid but with a small amount of β acid. The first fraction is suitable for adding to beer in very small quantities to improve the hop-like aroma. In contrast, the second is suitable for addition to the wort kettle. Finally, the third fraction is a possible starting point for what is called isomerised extract and is described below.

It has already been mentioned that α acids isomerise during boiling to more soluble and bitter compounds called iso α acids. The isomerisation can also be achieved by alkali treatment (e.g. sodium carbonate) to a solution of α acids or by heating solid material with catalysts such as magnesium salts. Unfortunately any contamination with β acids has to be rectified because they are substantially less soluble than iso α acids. The β acids can be precipitated by raising pH levels to 8.5 but of course the pH must be restored to around 5.0 in order to stabilise the iso α acids. Such isomerised extracts are suitable for adding directly to beer. Losses of bitter substances incurred during wort boiling and fermentation are avoided. Although isomerised extracts may be used to provide the bulk of the beer's bitterness, it is more usual to add the extracts to beer bittered normally so as to raise the bitterness levels to specification.

There are some beers that are packaged in clear glass bottles. When

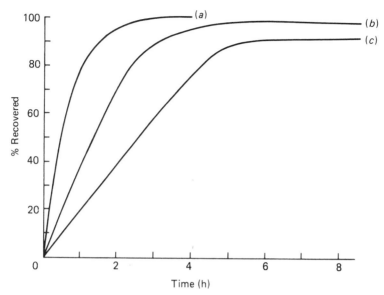

Fig. 6.10. The progressive extraction of essential oils and resins of hops during the liquid carbon dioxide process (*a*) essential oils, (*b*) β acids, (*c*) α acids.

packages of this kind are inadvertently exposed to sunlight, the iso α acids react with sulphur compounds present in the beer to yield an objectionable 'sun-struck' flavour aroma caused by the substance 3-methyl-2-butene-1-thiol. In order to prevent this reaction, isomerised extracts are used that have been chemically reduced. (The carbonyl group in the isohexanoyl sidechain is reduced by sodium borohydride to a secondary alcohol group.)

Extracts in general are advantageous compared with cone hops in taking up far less storage space, being relatively stable when stored at ambient temperature, permitting blending of hop varieties as required and allowing advantage to be taken of hops in larger quantities when the market price is low.

Wort boiling

The principal effects of wort boiling are:

(*a*) arrest of enzyme activity,
(*b*) sterilisation of the wort,
(*c*) coagulation of proteins and tannins,
(*d*) further precipitation of calcium phosphate and consequent fall in pH level,
(*e*) distillation of volatile materials,

(*f*)   evaporation of water and therefore concentration of the wort,
(*g*)   colour production from caramelisation of sugars, melanoidin
         formation and oxidation of tannins (these reactions also produce
         attractive toffee, nutty and burnt flavours into the wort).

In nearly all cases, hops or hop products will be present so that
additional considerations are:

(*h*)   wort is bittered by hop resins,
(*i*)   the surface tension of wort is reduced by oils and resins,
(*j*)   essential oils and in some instances tannins are added to wort,
(*k*)   iso α acids improve beer foam but essential oils reduce foam retention.

Several other materials may be added to the kettle in addition to
hops, notably sugars or cereal syrups (see p. 68). These liquid adjuncts
may serve as a wort extender, an inexpensive source of extract, a
diluent of wort nitrogen, a flavour improver or as a means of
high-gravity brewing. Such liquid adjuncts normally have a specific
gravity of about 1.150.

A further addition to the kettle may be extracts of brown or red
seaweeds. These alginates are polygalactose molecules that are strongly
sulphated and therefore highly negatively charged (Fig. 6.11). They will
therefore tend to coagulate positively charged proteins and thus increase
the weight of hot break or trub produced during the boil. A likely
consequence is that during cooling there will be less cold trub produced
which, because of its much smaller particles, is more difficult to remove
than hot trub. Even better, it is probable that there will be less tendency
for the beer to produce a haze after packaging. In some breweries the
kettle finings (clarifying agents), instead of being purified extracts, are
the dried entire seaweed – particularly the common British littoral red
seaweeds *Chondrus crispus* and *Gigartina stellata*.

The coagulation of proteins during boiling is very much influenced by
the presence of tannins and their composition, and also by the
combined effects of temperature, pH and multivalent ions such as
calcium and heavy metals. Heating causes the proteins to lose their
complex structure, to become uncoiled and to break at molecular
bridges to yield much smaller derivative molecules that should be called
polypeptides rather than proteins. The larger denatured molecules tend
to exceed their solubility limit, especially if close to their isoelectric
point. When they coagulate, often tanned by the malt and hop
polyphenols, hop resins tend to adsorb to them and so valuable hop
material is lost. Indeed it is common for only 30–50% of the α acid
material to be represented as iso α acids in the wort. The utilisation
falls to 20–40% by the time that beer goes into package.
Correspondingly there is a loss of wort nitrogen with trub formation,

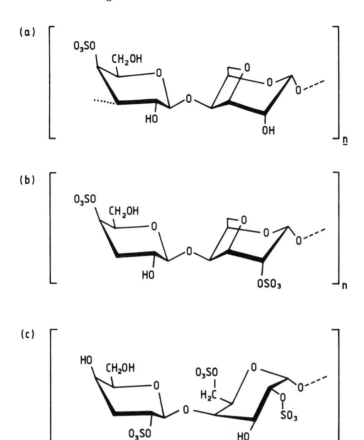

Fig. 6.11. The structures of (*a*) κ, (*b*) ι and (*c*) λ carageenans.

varying greatly but of the order of 50 mg l^{-1}. The trub takes the form of particles that are crudely spherical in shape, about 1 μm in diameter, and tending to associate to give flocs of up to 10 cm diameter.

The usual boil is for 60–90 min at atmospheric pressure (Fig. 6.12) but some brewers use pressure boiling and allow volatiles to escape at the end. Many will add a small proportion of their hops – the aroma hops with a delicate and attractive aroma – some 20 min before the end of the boil. In very recent years there has been the development of pressurised boiling at 140 °C for some 4 min. This not only saves time but with modern heat exchangers, is extremely economical in energy (Fig. 6.13). The use of steam in a traditional US brewery is shown in Fig. 6.14.

After the boil, the brewer clarifies the wort. If whole hops were used it would be necessary to sieve. The spent hops tend to form a filter bed

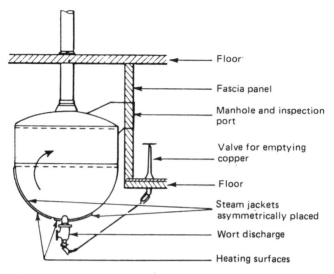

Fig. 6.12. A section of a typical brewery wort kettle.

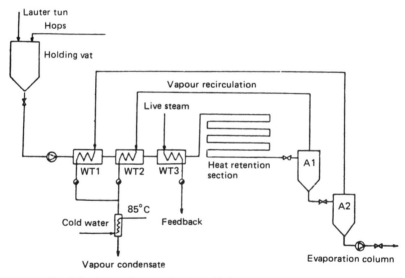

Fig. 6.13. A flow diagram showing a high pressure wort kettle (courtesy of Anton Steinecker GmbH, Freising, W. Germany). WT1, 2 and 3 are successive heat exchangers, raising the temperature to 140 °C. A1 and A2 permit loss of temperature and volatiles.

on which the trub accumulates. There is some value in this spent material as a garden fertiliser. The hops themselves serve as a mulch but it is the trub that makes dried hops a source of nitrogen, calcium, phosphorus and other mineral materials. Most brewers today use hops

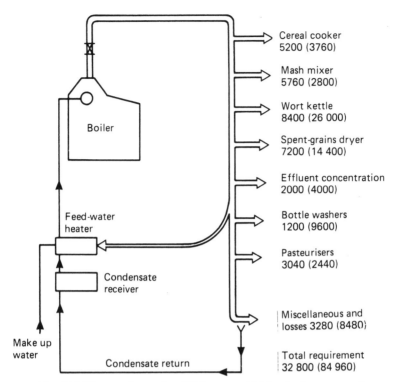

Fig. 6.14. The use of steam in a US brewery which has both a spent-grains dryer and effluent concentration. Each batch is 1000/hl at 14.5 °P over a 4/h cycle. The figures are the maximum load in kg/h⁻¹; those in brackets are total load for the batch in kg steam. After Fig. 18.5, *The Practical Brewer* published by the Master Brewers' Association of the Americas.

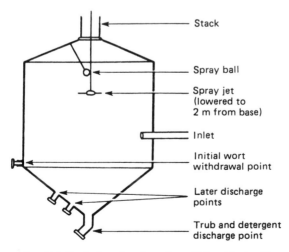

Fig. 6.15. Vertical section through a whirlpool tank with a conical base.

that have been ground just before use or as pellets. Instead of sieving, they clarify using a simple device called a whirlpool tank originally developed by the Molson breweries in Canada. A batch of wort is pumped at high speed (say 10 m s^{-1}) through a pipe set tangentially to the tank and possibly a third of the way up (Fig. 6.15). The circular momentum of the wort in the tank is soon replaced by one where the wort travels vertically down the walls and horizontally along the base to the centre, losing momentum by dragging against the tank wall. Solids in suspension are deposited as the wort slows, especially at the centre point of the base. The wort rises from the centre and repeats its circulatory path. After some 20–45 min, it is possible to withdraw clear wort from a suitable take-off point remote from the deposit of trub and hop material. The latter is often transferred to the spent grains.

Cooling and aeration

The early brewery-wort chillers were shallow vessels receiving a wort depth of perhaps 25 cm and situated at the top of the plant. Water vapour from the initially hot wort was permitted to escape through louvred openings. The same openings permitted air (laden with its normal complement of spores, pollen, insects and possibly industrial volatiles) to pass over the wort. Birds, attracted by the occasionally tropical environment, penetrated into the area and contaminated the wort with excrement (and, occasionally, dead bodies). On the positive side, the open vessels permitted not only cooling of the wort but also its aeration, helped by the large surface area exposed. Because of the shallow depth, particles of hot and cold trub settled.

Later chillers, developed for both dairies and breweries, permitted wort to flow as a thin film over a series of refrigerated pipes. Thus the

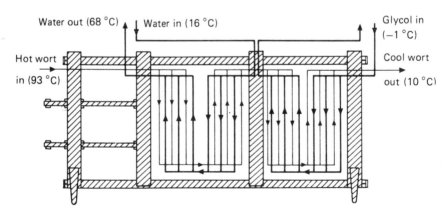

Fig. 6.16. Vertical section through a two-stage plate heat exchanger for cooling wort.

wort was chilled and aerated but clarification of the trub did not occur at this stage. Almost all breweries now employ enclosed-plate heat exchangers (Fig. 6.18). These comprise many plates of stainless steel, so indented by mechanical pressing that between each sheet is a shallow cavity. Wort passes from the first cavity to the cavity next but one and continues to alternate. Coolant, such as water runs counter-current to the wort. It therefore passes from the last cavity to the next but one. The wort and water streams are so arranged that they occupy alternate cavities. Thus wort at say 85 °C passes into the plate heat exchanger and emerges at 15 °C. Water enters the exchanger at 10 °C and, after cooling the wort, emerges at 75–80 °C. If the brewer requires wort at 10 °C, he arranges that the exchanger has a second section chilled with refrigerated water or alcohol or brine. Plate heat exchangers are very efficient in heat transfer but they are not primarily concerned with aeration and do nothing towards clarification. They are compact, hygienic and provide breweries with a large volume of water at 75–80 °C for cleaning purposes and possibly for mashing. (Water may also be heated by heat exchangers set in the wort kettle flues but this is less exploited.)

Aeration of wort is needed for yeast growth. Specifically it is required in small amounts (5–15 mg l^{-1}) by the cells in order to synthesise unsaturated fatty acids and sterols for intracellular membranes. If the requirements are at the lower end of the range, spraying wort into a fermenter may suffice. Most breweries will however introduce sterile air or oxygen into the wort stream in or near the heat exchanger. If injected into the hot wort entering the exchanger, the gas will only dissolve if it becomes chemically combined with wort constituents, for instance tannins. The turbulence in the exchanger aids the dissolving. Were the gas to be introduced into cool wort, it would dissolve physically. Air will provide a maximum of 8 mg l^{-1} dissolved oxygen. Some yeast strains however require more than this and oxygen is substituted for air. In order to exploit the turbulence of the exchanger, an ideal method is to introduce air or oxygen part way through the exchanger, for instance between the two stages. The wort then carries physically dissolved oxygen (and the wort darkening associated with oxidising tannins by hot aeration is avoided).

Removal of the cold trub is usually by settlement but there are breweries where it is filtered or centrifuged from the wort. One process involves pumping air into cold wort and removing the cold trub as a scum on the bubble froth. The wort is now ready for fermentation. In Britain, but in few other countries, the excise authorities make their measurements at this stage with the wort vulnerable to microbial infection. The volume of wort is gauged and its specific gravity (or original gravity, which is the technical term for wort gravity) is determined. Duty is paid on the product of volume and the difference between the specific gravities of the wort and water.

Comparison of substrate media for fermentation

Strains of the yeast *Saccharomyces* are used not only for fermenting brewers' wort but also a wide variety of other substrates (Table 6.5). In whisky production, the wort is not normally separated from the grains and is not boiled before yeast is added. Unhopped, unboiled but clarified wort is used to malt vinegar production; after fermentation the beer is acetified using specially selected acetic acid bacteria.

In cider and perry production, apples or pears are crushed and the juice extracted. The juice may be made microbiologically stable by additions of sulphur dioxide. For the production of red wine, grapes are crushed and fermented in the presence of sulphur dioxide. The skins, seeds and stalks are removed during the fermentation. In white wine manufacture, the grapes are crushed and the juice or must is clarified before fermentation in the presence of 100–200 mg l^{-1} of sulphur dioxide.

Table 6.5. *Typical analytical figures for brewers' wort, wine must and cider apple juice*

	Wort	Wine must	Cider apple juice
pH	5.0–5.6	2.7–3.3	3.3–4.0
SG	1.032–1.048	1.048–1.096	1.056
Glucose (% w/v)	0.8–1.0	6.5–12.0	1.5–2.0
Fructose (% w/v)	0.10–0.15	6.5–12.0	6.0
Sucrose (% w/v)	0.3–0.5	0.02–0.2	2.5–3.5
Maltose (% w/v)	3.3–5.4	–	–
Maltotriose (% w/v)	1.0–1.3	–	–
Organic acids (% w/v)	0.02	0.8–1.7 (especially malic and tartaric)	0.3–1.8 (malic most abundant)
Total nitrogen (mg l^{-1})	250–1100	300–1200	50–300
Free amino nitrogen (mg l^{-1})	160–300	250–1100	9–230
Total tannins (% w/v)	0.01–0.04	0.15–0.50	0.1–0.3

7 Yeasts and brewery bacteria

Simple classification of yeasts

Yeasts are unicellular budding fungi. They do not however fit neatly into one group of the fungi and therefore it is appropriate to outline the main divisions of the fungi in general.

Phycomycetes

Phycomycetes normally grow as mycelia; these are branched tubes (protected by a wall) of fairly uniform diameter which contain cytoplasm and numerous nuclei. The phycomycetal mycelia have no cross walls. Some (such as the bread moulds *Mucor* and *Rhizopus*) have male and female sex cells of the same size and shape. Others have larger female sex cells (e.g. *Pseudoperonospora*, the downy mildew of hops).

Ascomycetes

Ascomycetes have mycelia divided by cross walls; they have characteristic spores ('ascospores') which are produced in a sac called an ascus, after sexual fusion has occurred. Other spores that do not arise from sexual union are named conidia. This is the largest division of the fungi and includes many yeasts such as *Saccharomyces* and the moulds *Asperigillus* and *Penicillium* that are used extensively in microbiological industries.

Basidiomycetes

Basidiomycetes also have mycelia divided by cross walls but their basidiospores are formed in fours sprouting from a characteristic cell called a basidium. Rust and smut diseases of barley are examples of Basidiomycetes but mushrooms and toadstools are probably more familiar. Among the yeasts is the genus *Sporobolomyces* with unusual external shooting spores or ballistospores.

Fungi imperfecti

These represent the mixed bag of species whose sexual reproductive processes are unknown and where, therefore, characteristic spores do not arise. Occasionally a discovery is made of, for instance,

93

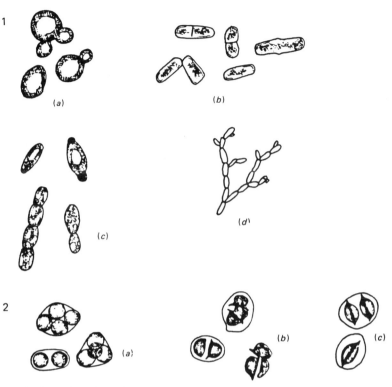

Fig. 7.1. 1. Drawings of (*a*) *Saccharomyces cerevisiae* (multilateral budding), (*b*) *Schizosaccharomyces pombe* (binary fission), (*c*) *Nadsonia* sp (bipolar budding), (d) pseudomycelium of *Pichia membranaefaciens*. 2. Asci and ascospores of (*a*) *Saccharomyces* sp, (*b*) *Pichia* sp and (*c*) *Hansenula saturnus*. Magnifications: mature cells of 1(*a*) are 8–10 μm in diameter and 1(*b*) and 1(*c*) are similar scale. 2(*a*), (*b*) and (*c*) are illustrated at twice the magnification of 1(*a*), (*b*) and (*c*); 1(*d*) is at half that magnification.

ascospores; the organism is then transferred to the Ascomycetes. Examples outside the yeasts include *Verticillium* wilt of hops and *Fusarium* infection of barley, but many yeasts are also included (such as *Candida* species).

Yeasts comprise some 39 genera and about 350 species. They are classified and identified partly on morphological and partly on physiological characteristics. Morphological aspects considered include the size and shape of cells in specified liquid and solid media, the mode of reproduction and whether the yeast forms a surface skin or a sediment in liquid media. Physiological characteristics are whether the yeast can grow on (and whether it can ferment) a particular carbohydrate, or whether it can utilise particular sources of nitrogen such as nitrate.

Yeast cells may be oval, spherical, lemon- or cigar-shaped. They may divide by budding from any position on the cell surface, or from the ends (or poles) of the cell only. Some do not bud although showing every other characteristic of yeasts; instead they form a cross wall within the cell after elongation. Particularly on solid media, some yeasts form branched or unbranched filaments, called pseudomycelia, instead of single cells; others form mycelia very similar to those of moulds (Fig. 7.1).

An example of physiological testing is that *Saccharomyces* species will not utilise nitrate as a source of nitrogen (although some genera such as *Hansenula* will). *Saccharomyces cerevisiae* can be distinguished from *S. carlsbergensis*, the other brewing species, because the former cannot ferment the sugar melibiose whereas the latter can. Both can use the sugar galactose but the yeast associated with sherry maturation, *S. bayanus* cannot. *S. capensis* does not ferment maltose but the other *Saccharomyces* species mentioned do.

Serological differentiation

One rapid method of distinguishing strains is based on serological techniques. It is invaluable in some instances but may be difficult to apply in others. Serological tests depend upon a very specific reaction between antibodies of mammalian blood and antigens (or foreign organic materials introduced into the blood). This is one of the key defence mechanisms of the human body; it copes successfully with bacterial infections and other foreign cells as well as large organic molecules.

Whole dead yeast cells (say strain A) are injected into an experimental animal, usually a rabbit. The animal produces antibodies with specific chemical groupings that complement those of the cell surface of the yeast which act as antigens. Following a course of injections, a volume of blood is withdrawn and is freed from red blood cells to yield a serum. This can be kept for long periods if stored cold in the presence of a preservative. When mixed with a suspension of the strain A yeast, the serum will agglutinate the cells; indeed it will agglutinate all strains that include on their surface one or more of the chemical groupings which acted as antigens.

Suppose that the serum (which is termed strain A antiserum) is treated with cells of a related strain B. The strain B will be agglutinated and use up antibodies that would react with both strains A and B. Were this repeated, the so-called absorbed antiserum would no longer have the antibodies to react with B but might well agglutinate strain A because there are probably chemical groupings or antigens on A not shared with B. This can be exploited as shown in Table 7.1 to indicate relationships between strains, or even species and genera. Alternatively, it can be used to identify unknown strains.

Table 7.1. *Agglutination of various Saccharomyces by using strain A_1 antiserum before and after absorption*

Yeast strains under test	Agglutination using unabsorbed serum	Agglutination after absorption with			
		A_1 or A_2 or A_3	B_1 or B_2 or B_3	C_1 or C_2	D_1 or D_2 or D_3
A_1, A_2, A_3 (*S. carlsbergensis*)	+	−	+	+	+
B_1, B_2, B_3 (*S. carlsbergensis*)	+	−	−	−	−
C_2, C_2 (*S. rouxii*)	+	−	+	−	+
D_1, D_2, D_3 (*S. cerevisiae*)	+	−	+	−	−

It is useful that antibodies may be coupled to fluorescent dyes because antibodies reacting with a specific yeast strain will make the yeast surface fluoresce. Much smaller quantities of antisera are needed to carry out tests than is the case with mass agglutination. With a suitable microscope and quartz-iodine illumination, it is possible to identify single fluorescing cells within thousands of non-fluorescing ones. It is therefore possible to identify the presence of unwanted yeast strains (called wild yeasts) in very low concentrations within a culture yeast – provided a suitable antiserum can be prepared which will react with the wild yeast but not the culture yeast. The extent that a cell fluoresces can be enhanced by a modification to the technique. The absorbed antiserum that is to be used for the work is, instead of being coupled to a dye, injected into a goat. Antiserum against the rabbit antiserum can then be prepared from the goat's blood. This is coupled with the dye. To detect the wild yeast, the absorbed antiserum is first added to the yeast suspension. It is followed by the fluorescent antisera from the goat. The wild yeast has a first coat of rabbit antiserum and a second coat of goat (anti-rabbit) antiserum. More dye molecules can be coated on the yeast than if the simpler single-coat technique is used.

Structure of the yeast cell

A typical brewing yeast cell will, when fully grown, be between 8 and 14 μm diameter and have a mass of about 40 pg when dry. Thus 10^{12} dried cells will weigh 40 g. In the living, pressed state, the same number of cells will weigh 200 g. Examination of yeast by a light microscope reveals that the cell is bounded by a wall; within the cell few structures can be distinguished except one or more vacuoles. Phase-contrast microscopy or stained preparations may be used to demonstrate the presence of a nucleus and various other organelles. The surface of yeast can be studied using scanning electron microscopy and internal structures by transmission electron microscopy on freeze-fractured preparations of fresh, unfixed cells. A diagram of a section of a typical brewing yeast is shown in Fig. 7.2. More detailed information on parts of the cell is obtained by biochemical identification of components.

The cell wall represents 30% of the total dry mass of the cell and is 100–200 nm thick. It comprises about 40% β glucans, 40% α mannans, 8% protein, 7% lipid, 3% inorganic material and 2% hexosamine and chitin. The glucan is linked to protein and represents the major structural component and is mainly on the inside of the wall. Mannan is also linked to the proteins, sometimes through the hexosamine, and tends to be on the outside of the walls. The surface of the cell is charged due to the presence of carboxyl and phosphate groupings which, at the pH of beer, confer a strong negative charge. Amino groupings are also present but only confer local regions of positive charge. Cell walls can be dissolved by a mixed-enzyme preparation from an actinomycete called *Arthrobacter luteus* or from the digestive gland of the edible snail, *Helix pomatia*. Usually, a reducing agent such as mercaptoethanol is also required. If the yeast cells are held in an osmotic stabiliser, such as a 20% aqueous solution of mannitol, the cells remain intact but spherical after losing their walls. They are now called spheroplasts and will, given appropriate growth conditions, resynthesise their walls. This is exploited in certain techniques for the genetic manipulation of yeast.

The yeast cell multiplies by budding. A weakened area of the wall permits the cytoplasm to bulge out and the new bud surface is immediately provided with a wall. As the bud grows, organelles from the mother cell migrate to it, including a nucleus (after the mother nucleus has divided). Eventually the bud is fully grown but may not necessarily detach. It is quite common for yeasts to form large chains of cells because of non-disjunction. If the cell does break away, the mother's cell wall has a raised ring of material called a bud-scar while the corresponding birth-scar on the bud is less easily distinguished. More than 30 buds may be produced from a single cell during its lifetime but is rare for more than two or three to be present at any one time.

Enzymes secreted from the yeast cell penetrate the cell wall. The most notable is invertase which hydrolyses sucrose before it diffuses into the cell. Acid phosphatase is also present. *Saccharomyces carlsbergensis* secretes melibiase, but not the related *Saccharomyces cerevisiae*. Some yeasts secrete proteases in appreciable amount but *Saccharomyces* species have only a limited activity in this respect.

The boundary of the cytoplasm is a living membrane, the

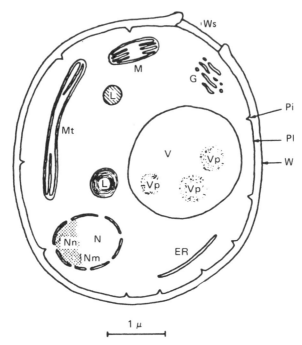

Fig. 7.2. Diagram of an electron micrograph of a section through a resting cell of bakers' yeast (*Saccharomyces cerevisiae*). ER, endoplastic reticulum; M, mitochondrion; N, nucleus; Nm, nuclear membrane; Nn, nucleolus; Pi, invagination; Pl, plasmalemma; V, vacuole; Vp, polymetaphosphate granule; W, cell wall; Ws, bud-scar; L, lipid granule (sphaerosome).

plasmalemma. It not only covers the cytoplasm, it ramifies it by joining up with the internal network of membranes. These structures comprise lipid, phospholipid, protein and sterols. The plasmalemma is important in regulating the flow of all materials in and out of the cell. Other membranes probably compartmentalise the cell and also provide a surface on which certain enzymes operate.

The nucleus of the yeast is about 1.5 μm diameter and is bounded by a double membrane. A dense crescent-shaped area within it is called the nucleolus. Chromosomes are not discernible but genetic evidence for *Saccharomyces cerevisiae* indicates that there are at least 17 pairs and several fragments in the diploid cells (see p. 99).

Rapidly growing yeast cells may have several vacuoles but the mature cell normally has one. Within its single membrane are dense particles of polyphosphate which are traditionally called volutin granules. When yeast cells grow under aerobic conditions and particularly when glucose concentrations are low, several mitochondria are present in each cell. The mitochondria, each bounded by a double membrane, provide sites for the cytochromes and respiratory enzymes and for the generation of adenosine triphosphate (ATP). Thus they are responsible for the oxidative metabolism of sugars to carbon dioxide and water; the ATP they generate represents the chemical energy derived from these reactions. Under anaerobic conditions or when glucose concentrations are high, the mitochondria appear to atrophy and lose their biochemical abilities, at least temporarily. The changes can readily be monitored by observing the cytochrome spectrum of the yeast. An aerobic yeast has a four-banded spectrum while an anaerobically growing yeast has only two bands.

The cell wall in brewing

Differences in the chemical structure of the outer layers of the yeast cell wall lead to some strains rising to the top of the fermenting wort towards the end of fermentation. These 'top yeasts' contrast with 'bottom yeasts' that tend to sink to the base of the fermentor. The distinction can be simulated in water; top yeasts, but not bottom yeasts, tend to be somewhat hydrophobic and collect at the meniscus. In traditional fermentations, somewhat different processing is necessary for the two types of yeast.

Some yeast strains have buds which only sever from the mother cell with difficulty. Chains of many cells therefore develop and are able to settle more quickly unless they are buoyed by a bubble of carbon dioxide. Other strains have the quite distinct characteristic of being flocculent. Individual cells are attracted to each other to form a floc, possibly comprising thousands or even millions of cells. The attraction is thought to be partly due to the bridging by calcium ions of carboxyl groups on adjacent cells brought together by mixing currents, and partly by hydrogen bonding between the cells. Flocculent strains settle more readily then non-flocculent or powdery strains and the two types have been exploited in different kinds of fermentor (see Chapter 8).

Yeast life cycle

Most yeast strains exist in the 'diplophase', that is the cells contain two sets of chromosomes. This condition is maintained as the yeast multiplies by budding. Particularly under adverse conditions, however, certain cells may become asci and each forms ascospores.

An ascospore has only a single set of chromosomes. During the reduction division which occurs within the nucleus in order to arrive at the 'haplophase' condition, there is a segregation of genetic material (Fig. 7.3). For instance if one of a pair of chromosomes of the diploid mother cell has a dominant gene for fermentation of the sugar galactose

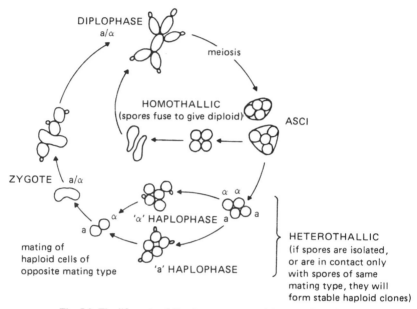

Fig. 7.3. The life cycle of *Saccharomyces cerevisiae*: a and α refer to the genes controlling the mating response.

and the other has (at the corresponding locus) a recessive allele which does not code for the enzyme dealing with galactose), then one daughter cell receives the dominant gene while the other daughter cell receives the recessive. Generally, this reduction division (or meiosis) is followed by one or more divisions that do not reduce chromosome number further, so that the ascus eventually contains four or eight haploid ascospores. If all the ascospores were to survive and propagate (and such an eventuality is rare), then half of the ascospores would be able to ferment galactose and half would not.

Let us take a further instance, where a second pair of chromosomes carries the gene for the synthesis of leucine on one of the pair and the corresponding recessive gene (which does not provide for this synthesis) is on the other chromosome. During reduction division, not only will the galactose genes segregate, so also will the leucine genes. The ascospores produced will comprise 25% with both dominant genes, 25% with both recessive genes, 25% with dominant galactose gene but recessive leucine gene and finally 25% with recessive galactose and dominant leucine gene.

In brewing yeast, ascospores are not set free from the ascus and instead fuse within it to produce the diplophase condition again before the ascus wall breaks. Physical separation of the ascospores by the microbiologist cutting the ascus wall is therefore necessary in order to investigate the genetic make-up of each ascospore. There are two general types of yeast with respect to isolated ascospore development. Some, called 'homothallic', have ascospores which will germinate and divide to form two haploid cells, which will promptly fuse to reestablish the diplophase. Others, called 'heterothallic', have ascospores which only fuse with the opposite mating type. Thus a heterothallic diplophase cell will contain genes for both mating types; half of the ascospores will have the one mating gene, and half the other. Incredibly, the two mating types are referred to as a and α.

Selection of yeast strains

It has been relatively easy to develop new strains of yeast for bread making. It was discovered that at least some of the strains propagated specially for baking easily sporulated, were heterothallic and yielded a high proportion of viable ascospores. It was therefore possible to hybridise, under controlled conditions, two haploid cells of choice. This situation contrasts markedly from that of brewing yeasts, which sporulate with difficulty and produce few viable ascospores. The bakers have exploited the situation by seeking hybrids that grow quickly in propagators, store well as a slab of yeast cake and rapidly ferment when added to bread dough. Brewers' requirements, especially those relating to beer flavour, are far more complex; therefore genetic manipulation of brewing yeasts is a phenomenon of the 1980s, some 25–30 years later than the successful application of yeast genetics to bakers' yeast.

The brewer requires primarily a yeast that will yield a beer of desirable flavour and aroma. Only in the last 10 years has it been possible to quantify aspects of flavour and aroma sufficiently for brewers to provide even an elementary specification. It is complicated because flavour and aroma are derived partly from the raw materials and processing and partly from the metabolism of the yeast. Thus the levels of diacetyl (which imparts the flavour and aroma of butterscotch) are influenced by the raw materials, wort-production methods, the yeast, the fermentation and post-fermentation conditions and, finally, by the infection of the beer by various bacteria and wild yeasts.

Another requirement of the brewers is that the yeast grows adequately. Clearly, the brewer requires a sufficient crop to propagate the yeast effectively – usually a 3–5-fold increase during a fermentation. Less than this causes operating difficulties, but too much means that excessive amounts of carbohydrate that might have been transformed into ethanol have been incorporated into yeast biomass. A brewer does not get a sufficient return from selling his surplus yeast to countenance over-production.

The ability of a yeast to form flocs or to rise to the top of the fermentor have been important characteristics in fermentation systems employed in the past. However, the tendency for most large breweries to adopt similar kinds of large fermentor has meant a change in emphasis. Particularly for the large brewery, there is interest in how well the yeast separates from the beer in the base of the fermentor. It will be appreciated that this, in common with the other requirements mentioned above are not easily quantified. The brewer has to select on the basis of small-scale fermentations, but even with these, the results are quantitatively different (and sometimes qualitatively different) from vessels of 20 l, 20 hl and 2000 hl.

Maintenance of yeast cultures

It is possible to separate individual cells one from other by the process of micromanipulation, that is using a microscopic glass rod to push and pull cells to separate drops of water so that they can be picked up by sterile slivers of filter paper and dropped into separate bottles of sterile growth medium. This technique might be applied to a mixture of yeasts or to a contaminated yeast culture. It would then be necessary to select the yeast required from the collection. A less rigorous but simpler method is to streak a culture of the mixed or contaminated yeast onto a petri dish containing sterile solidified growth medium. After colonies had grown, certain ones would be picked off and then streaked again onto a fresh dish. The new lot of colonies, when grown, would be the collection used for the selection of the replacement yeast.

Yeast cultures may be held at room temperature on slopes of solidified growth medium or in liquid culture at about 4 °C. In order to maintain more anaerobic conditions, it is possible to pour sterile mineral oil over the culture. Ascospore formation should be avoided.

In general, freeze-drying (or lyophilisation) has not been very successful in maintaining brewing yeasts. The viability tends to be very low and those cells surviving may well be mutants. Considerable success has been claimed however for storing in a glycerol–serum medium, held in a sealed vial and submerged in liquid nitrogen (-196 °C).

When a yeast is required for brewing, the culture is propagated in 10 ml of sterilised brewers' wort and this is used for the inoculum for 2 l of the same medium. This volume is sufficient to seed a modern yeast propagator of say 50 hl capacity. Such a propagator (Fig. 7.4) would be kept rigorously free of infection and the culture would be aerated intermittently with sterile air in such a way that foaming was not excessive. The whole culture would be used to inoculate a full-scale fermenter of 500 hl, usually while the yeast was in logarithmic phase of growth (Fig. 7.5) and fermentation incomplete.

Propagation of yeasts in breweries contrasts strongly with the method

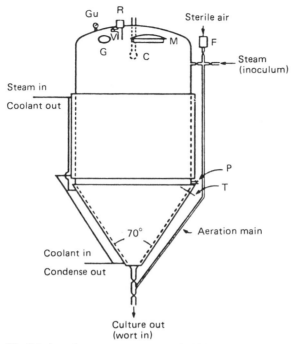

Fig. 7.4. A modern yeast propagator of 50 hl capacity. C, sprayball for cleaning; F, secondary air filter; G, sight glass; Gu, pressure gauge; M, manway; P, sample point; R, pressure/vacuum relief valve with air-sterilising filter; T, temperature probe; V, vent with shut-off valve.

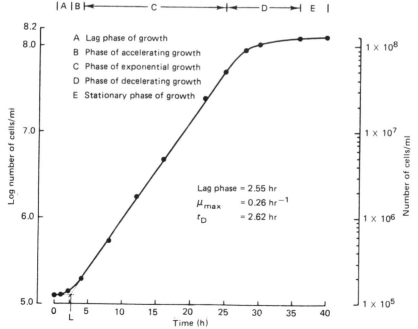

A Lag phase of growth
B Phase of accelerating growth
C Phase of exponential growth
D Phase of decelerating growth
E Stationary phase of growth

Lag phase = 2.55 hr
μ_{max} = 0.26 hr^{-1}
t_D = 2.62 hr

Fig. 7.5. Phases of growth of a yeast in batch culture. μ_{max} is the maximum specific growth rate and t_D is the doubling time.

employed for bakers' yeast. For the latter, it is important to avoid any fermentation and to use the carbohydrate as effectively as possible in producing yeast biomass. It has been discovered that this is best achieved by providing an excess of sterile air and maintaining a low level of nutrients. If the carbohydrate in the feed were above say 0.1%, there would be an opportunity for fermentation. Instead, the carbohydrate (in the form of molasses) is fed at logarithmically increasing rates to just keep pace with yeast growth. This process yields 100 g dry mass of yeast for every 200 g of sucrose used. In comparison, the same weight of carbohydrate would yield one tenth the weight of yeast in a brewery fermentor but almost 100 g of ethanol.

Wild yeasts

Unwanted yeasts in breweries are called 'wild'. Some are strains of *Saccharomyces cerevisiae*, or strains of other species of the same genus, or belong to such genera as *Candida*, *Pichia*, *Hansenula* or *Torulopsis*. Most have the ability to produce abnormal flavours and aromas, to produce turbidity that is difficult to remove from beer and some will develop pellicles at the surface of the beer.

Elimination of wild yeasts or holding numbers low is usually a matter of using a clean pitching yeast in the brewery, possibly by repropagating from laboratory stocks every 1–2 months. Equipment must be clean and sterile. Microbiological checks for wild yeasts and contaminating bacteria are made on cooled worts, sterile air lines, pitching yeast and any materials being added to beer. The serological test referred to earlier is often used for wild yeasts of the genus *Saccharomyces*. Others not in this genus may be detected by a series of tests such as their ability to grow on a medium with the amino acid lysine as sole nitrogen source, their ability to withstand – better than culture yeasts – higher concentrations of the antibiotic actidione (cycloheximide) or the dye crystal violet or the dye derivative fuchsin sulphite.

Two types of *S. cerevisiae* wild yeasts call for comment. The first is a group of yeasts that have lost the ability to switch to aerobic metabolism from fermentative metabolism because of various mutations. These respiratory-deficient yeasts survive alongside culture yeasts and are claimed to produce abnormal flavours and aromas, including the precursor of diacetyl. They may also be recognised by their inability (unlike brewing yeast) to use glycerol as a carbon source. A second group has the ability to secrete a protein that will destroy the plasma membranes of susceptible yeasts and therefore kill them. Brewing yeasts are commonly sensitive to these zymocidal proteins, so their producers are serious contaminants. Fortunately the zymocide is effective only over a narrow range of pH. It is only, therefore, in the continuous fermentation processes (which maintain such a pH range indefinitely) where the entire culture yeast may be eliminated and where the wild yeast can take over rapidly and produce beer with off flavours.

Applications of yeast genetics in producing new strains

It is possible to obtain yeasts with different characteristics by irradiation with ultraviolet light or the use of chemical mutagens. The changes occur because of random damage to the chromosomes and therefore it is rare that a desirable new feature arises without loss of desirable characters that previously existed. Classical genetics of brewing yeasts is difficult because of poor ability to produce viable ascospores and reluctance of the haploids to fuse. Nevertheless this can sometimes be achieved by the technique of rare-mating. As an example, one parent might be a culture with respiratory deficiency but able to grow on a medium containing ammonium salts as the sole source of nitrogen. The other parent would be respiratory sufficient but with a requirement for the amino acid leucine. Neither parent would grow on a medium lacking leucine and having glycerol as a carbon source. Any hybrid of the two would be able to do so and could be recognised even if it were the sole one in a million cells on a petri dish.

One example of rare-mating and a process called cytoduction being successfully applied is shown in Fig. 7.6. Mention is made above of yeasts that secrete zymocides. A brewing strain doing so would be advantageous in killing at least a proportion of any contaminating yeasts that were present during fermentation. A parent of the strain is a brewing yeast capable of using ammonium salt as the sole source of nitrogen and with a respiratory deficiency associated with the cytoplasm, in fact with the mitochondrial DNA. The other parent is a haploid strain with the ability to produce zymocide determined by cytoplasmic RNA. It also has a gene which causes failure of the nuclei of a hybrid cell to fuse and requires histidine for growth. The medium used to select progeny is devoid of histidine and would support the growth of only respiratory-sufficient cells. Some 5–180 zygotes are produced for each 10^8 cells used. Because of the gene hindering nuclear fusion, some of the zygotes have nuclei identical with the brewing yeast but have acquired the cytoplasmic genes for zymocide production and respiratory sufficiency.

A further method of carrying out genetic manipulation of yeast is to dissolve away the cell walls of the two prospective parent strains. This is achieved by suspending yeasts in an osmotic stabiliser, either a solution of mannitol or more commonly sorbitol. The walls are digested by either a β glucuronidase enzyme preparation from the digestive

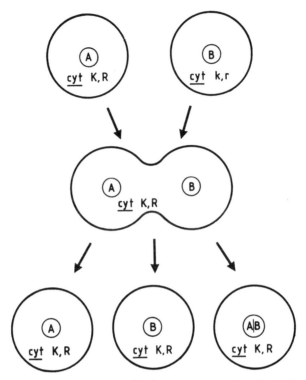

Fig. 7.6. Fusion of a haploid laboratory yeast and a polyploid brewing yeast to yield a brewing yeast with special characters. The haploid nucleus (A) has a dominant gene that confers an inability of the nucleus to fuse with another yeast nucleus and recessive genes that confer a nutritional requirement for adenine and histidine. Cytoplasmic genes include one that codes for killer protein and another for respiratory normality. In contrast the brewing yeast has dominant nuclear genes that confer the ability to synthesise adenine and histidine plus recessive cytoplasmic genes for respiratory deficiency (the yeast will not grow on glycerol) and for killer character. On a glycerol medium free of adenine and histidine, about one cell in a million grows and this must be due to fusion of the two types of cell. The nuclei themselves rarely fuse. Products of the cell fusion include the one in the middle of the bottom row which has the brewing yeast nucleus but with cytoplasmic genes for respiratory normality and killer character.

gland of the Roman snail or a β glucanase preparation from the microorganism *Arthrobacter luteus*. In one experiment one parent was *Saccharomyces cerevisiae* which failed to sporulate, and which fermented maltose (but not lactose); the other was the yeast *Kluyveromyces lactis* which also fails to sporulate and ferments lactose (but not maltose). The product from fusing the spheroplasts (in the presence of polyethylene glycol and calcium ions) was a hybrid capable of sporulating and of fermenting both lactose and maltose. The walls of the hybrid were restored by embedding the spheroplasts in a nutrient medium solidified with 3% agar.

A further method also involves using spheroplasts of one strain. This is the yeast that will receive nucleic acid material from the donor strain. Cells of the latter are broken up and the chromosomal material is separated. Enzymes are used to break up the yeast chromosomes into short lengths and this is incorporated into what are termed plasmid vectors. The vectors are often circular chromosomes found in bacteria such as *Escherichia coli* or in the cytoplasm of yeast. Such vectors readily penetrate into spheroplasts and operate speparately from the chromosomal complement of the recipient strain. In one instance the recipient strain would only grow in the presence of leucine but, after transfer of donor material carrying the gene for leucine synthesis, the transformed recipient was capable of growing on a medium free from leucine.

These various techniques are at present being used to produce brewing yeasts that have the ability to ferment dextrins, that is products of the digestion of starch that are too large to be fermented by normal brewing strains. Conferring such an ability upon a brewing yeast means that it would be able to ferment wort to completion, instead of leaving some 20% unfermented. At present this aim is only achieved by adding a fungal enzyme called amyloglucosidase to the fermenting wort. The product is called 'light' or 'lite' beer. Labelling laws may demand disclosure of the enzyme addition.

A further aim is to provide brewing yeast with the ability to degrade β glucan gums that may cause difficulty with wort and beer clarification. Such enzymes are present in certain moulds and bacteria. Attempts to insert the gene into yeast may have been successful but unfortunately the gene conferring β glucanase activity has not as yet expressed itself to a demonstrable extent. Other work is attempting to insert into brewing yeast genes conferring strong proteolytic activity. This might have the advantage of degrading those proteins which produce a haze when beer is chilled. There is also interest in yeasts that are able to produce less of the precursor of the diketone diacetyl – a substance which has a pronounced butterscotch flavour. (Yeast does not produce the diketone directly, it secretes the precursor which is chemically transformed in the medium to diacetyl; yeast is then able to chemically reduce the diacetyl – but often incompletely – to a virtually tasteless substance, 2,3 butanediol.)

In conclusion, it is interesting to note that yeasts have been modified by the use of plasmid vectors to produce successfully a range of mammalian products including the antiviral agent interferon, the hormone insulin and a bovine growth hormone.

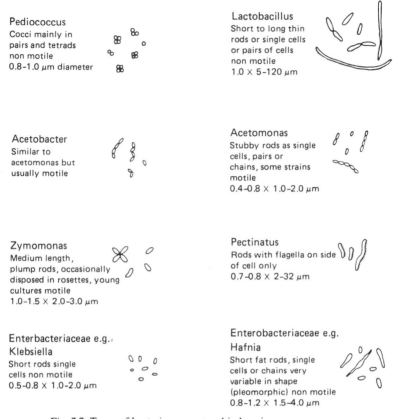

Pediococcus
Cocci mainly in
pairs and tetrads
non motile
0.8-1.0 μm diameter

Lactobacillus
Short to long thin
rods or single cells
or pairs of cells
non motile
1.0 × 5-120 μm

Acetobacter
Similar to
acetomonas but
usually motile

Acetomonas
Stubby rods as single
cells, pairs or
chains, some strains
motile
0.4-0.8 × 1.0-2.0 μm

Zymomonas
Medium length,
plump rods, occasionally
disposed in rosettes, young
cultures motile
1.0-1.5 × 2.0-3.0 μm

Pectinatus
Rods with flagella on side
of cell only
0.7-0.8 × 2-32 μm

Enterbacteriaceae e.g.
Klebsiella
Short rods single
cells non motile
0.5-0.8 × 1.0-2.0 μm

Enterobacteriaceae e.g.
Hafnia
Short fat rods, single
cells or chains very
variable in shape
(pleomorphic) non motile
0.8-1.2 × 1.5-4.0 μm

Fig. 7.7. Types of bacteria encountered in brewing.

Bacteria that contaminate wort and beer

Wort is a comparatively rich medium but this is boiled and, after very little delay, is inoculated with yeast. During fermentation, the pH falls from about 5.3 to 4.1, ethanol is produced to a value of 3–4% w/v and there is a substantial fall in the concentrations of sugars, amino acids and vitamins. Beer is therefore a relatively poor medium for bacterial growth and the range of bacteria that commonly contaminate is small. As with wild yeast infections, there is often turbidity of the beer and abnormal flavours and aromas.

Lactic acid bacteria are the only Gram-positive bacteria that cause serious problems in the brewery environment. Two genera are commonly encountered; *Lactobacillus* species have rod-shaped cells and *Pediococcus* species have spherical ones (Fig. 7.7). From a physiological point of view, the lactic acid bacteria fall into two groups, the

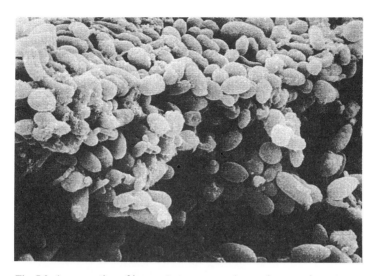

Fig. 7.8. A preparation of brewers' yeast seen under an electron microscope. Each yeast cell is about 8–10 microns in length. A few rod-shaped bacteria contaminates the yeast. The amorphous coating on some yeasts is precipitated beer protein.

thermophiles and the mesophiles. Lactic acid bacteria can also be divided from a biochemical standpoint into those which produce lactic acid as their principal metabolic product and those that yield, in addition, a variety of products (including acetic acid). Fig. 7.8 shows a few rod-shaped contaminants in a brewers' yeast preparation.

Some German breweries, keeping to the spirit of the Beer Purity Laws, need to break down bicarbonate not with the addition of mineral acid but by encouraging thermophilic lactic acid bacteria to grow on the mash and produce lactic acid. Indeed in many foods and beverages, lactic acid bacteria are encouraged to sour the material; examples include cheeses, yoghurt, American sour whisky, sauerkraut, pickled vegetables and sour-dough bread. In wine making, particularly in Portugal, the semi-sparkling condition arises from lactic acid bacteria attacking malic acid of the grape juice to yield lactic acid and carbon dioxide.

Lactic acid bacteria are serious contaminants of beer and are important producers of unwanted metabolites including the precursor of butterscotch-flavoured diacetyl. They are difficult to eradicate but it is surprising how difficult it sometimes is to isolate and grow them in the laboratory. Once isolated, they require for growth a medium which is neutral, rich in amino acids and in vitamins. A carbon dioxide atmosphere may be needed. Once growing, it is often difficult (if not impossible) to wean them back onto beer.

Turning now to Gram-negative bacteria, probably the most important are what are called wort bacteria. These belong to the family Enterobacteriaceae which includes many bacteria associated with either vegetable matter or the gut of many animals, *Escherichia coli* being the most familiar example. There are two general types that grow in wort. The first grows well until, due to the fermentative activities of yeast, the pH of the fermenting wort falls to about 4.4 and the alcohol levels rise to about 2% w/v. At this stage, genera such as *Enterobacter* and *Citrobacter* die but the products of their metabolism are left in the beer, often giving rise to abnormal flavours and aromas. The second group survives the fermentation and are harvested along with the yeast. They are therefore transferred to subsequent fermentations. Such bacteria (*Hafnia*, *Obesumbacterium*) have metabolic abilities similar to those of yeast but cause abnormal flavours and aromas such as excessive production of volatile sulphur compounds. They may cause beer pH to be higher than normal, may restrict the growth of yeast and, in general, adjust the environment for their own better survival.

Acetic acid bacteria are familiar acetifying organisms. They are used commercially for producing vinegar from wine, cider or unhopped malt beer. Similarly, with beer left exposed to air, they oxidise the alcohol to acetic acid. This used to be common with traditional draught ale but better standards of hygiene have reduced its incidence. Nevertheless these bacteria are common contaminants of pipes from keg or cask to the bar tap, even when pasteurised keg beer is being passed through the lines.

Other Gram-negative bacteria encountered in breweries include the genus *Zymomonas*, common in the sweetened beer in the UK. This produces excessive quantities of acetaldehyde and hydrogen sulphide, an objectionable mixture originally given the name 'Burton stench'. In recent years another genus, *Pectinatus* has been discovered growing in sterile-filtered beer in bottles under anaerobic conditions and producing a range of metabolites including butyric acid. Other genera, including the Gram-positive spore formers *Bacillus* and *Clostridium*, are encountered in small numbers in beer. It could be that they are chance contaminants that survive but do not grow. But brewery microbiologists must be ready for the unexpected contaminants.

It is often necessary to count bacteria in the presence of a large yeast population. This is achieved by incorporating the antibiotic actidione (or cycloheximide) at 10 ppm into the growth medium, an effective way of inhibiting yeast growth. To count individual groups of bacteria it is necessary to develop selective media, i.e. media which will support the growth of one group but not another. For example, acetic acid bacteria will grow on a medium where ethanol is the sole source of carbon; most other brewery bacteria will fail to grow. The selective media are used in the solidified form in petri dishes. A sample bacterial suspension is spread over the surface of the medium and the number of colonies that develop indicates the number of viable cells present in the sample.

Control of infection

Yeast used to inoculate brewers' wort is an important reservoir of infections. Some breweries will keep down bacterial infection by periodic washing of the yeast with mineral acid, usually at about pH 2.5. The time and temperature regime of the washing is critical otherwise the bacteria are not killed or, at the other extreme, the yeast is killed by the treatment. Other breweries prefer to discard their yeast after using it for say 10–12 fermentations in sequence and replace it with a freshly propagated culture.

Brewery equipment is commonly constructed of austenitic stainless steel, which is easy to clean. There has also been a tendency to use more and more totally enclosed vessels, thereby almost eliminating air-borne infection. Sanitising vessels and other stainless steel equipment is now reasonably standardised. The sequence is wash thoroughly by water, using high pressure revolving jets or static spray balls in the vessels. When the water has drained, hot caustic soda (usually with some sodium hypochlorite) is used as a detergent-sanitiser. The caustic soda kills microbes effectively and is an excellent dissolver of protein. It is not however suitable for dissolving and keeping in suspension calcium salts, therefore additions of various polyphosphates, metasilicates or gluconates may be made (Table 7.2). The hypochlorite is a source of free chlorine and therefore a strong bacteriocide; it also enhances the cleaning power of the detergent. Free chlorine is however a dangerous agent of corrosion of stainless steel if the pH of the solution falls to neutrality or below.

Some breweries use the detergent sanitiser once only and then discharge to drain, others reuse it and maintain the level of causticity which will fall particularly if carbon dioxide is present. After the detergent-sanitising, it is necessary to wash again but with sterile water and to ensure that all detergent-sanitiser has been removed from the surfaces. This rinse water can be reused as the first rinse water.

The cost of manpower is high and therefore many breweries, and particularly large ones, use automated controls for the washing sequences and recyclings. Microprocessors are presently being applied to this operation which is called 'Cleaning in place' (or CIP).

Some of the vessels cleaned contain carbon dioxide and are situated in cold rooms. There is therefore interest in using in such vessels a cold

Table 7.2. *Properties of components of commercial cleaning mixtures*[a]

	Organic dissolving power (wort beer and yeast residues)	Wetting power (penetration of detergents)	Dispersing power (hold insoluble particles of dirt in suspension)	Rinsing power	Germicidal power	Calcium sequestering power (keep carbonate in solution)	Calcium dissolving power (dissolve calcium salts in alkaline solution)
Caustic soda	5	1	1	1	3		
Sodium carbonate	2	1	1	1	1		
Sodium metasilicate	3	3	4	3	2		
Sodium orthosilicate	3	2	4	3	3		
Trisodium phosphate	2	2	4	3	2		
Wetting agents		5	4	5			
Sodium tripolyphosphate	2	1	3	2		3	
Sodium hexametaphosphate			4	2		4	1
Ethylene diamine tetraacetic acid						5	5
Sodium gluconate						5	3

[a] The strength of various properties is indicated by a scale in which 5 is the maximum strength. Mixtures of caustic soda, sodium metasilicate, wetting agent, and sodium tripolyphosphate will cover most requirements. EDTA and gluconates are included for mixtures required to remove beerstone and heater-scale, the former in acidic and weakly alkaline solutions, the latter in alkaline solutions.

detergent-sanitiser which is not based on caustic soda. Alternatively, nitrogen is being used as a substitute for carbon dioxide in vessels that need to be free of oxygen.

Microbiological control involves taking samples frequently from many brewery locations. The surfaces to be examined may be wiped with sterile swabs and the latter washed in sterile growth medium. Microbial growth in the medium indicates a contaminated surface. Wort or beer samples may be withdrawn through sample taps, or by using a hypodermic syringe through rubber septa in the vessel or pipe surface.

Breweries should be and frequently are extremely hygienic locations. They should match the best dairies in this respect.

8   Fermentation – the fundamental process

Wort – the rich medium

Hopped wort made available to yeast in a brewery fermenter is a rich medium (Table 8.1). It contains assimilable carbohydrate, a wide range of amino acids and other simple nitrogenous materials, mineral salts including calcium, magnesium, sodium, potassium, iron, zinc, copper and manganese, chloride, sulphate, carbonate and phosphate. Vitamins such as biotin, pantothenic acid, inositol, thiamin, pyridoxine and nicotinic acid are present.

Yeast requires these simple sugars, amino acids, salts and vitamins to grow. Additionally it needs sterols, unsaturated fatty acids and dissolved oxygen. Apart from the oxygen and some of the salts, malt (and adjuncts, if used) furnishes the rest of the requirements. The sugars provide for energy production and for biosynthesis, the amino acids for biosynthesis (especially of proteins), while the salts and vitamins play important metabolic roles. Membrane synthesis depends on unsaturated fatty acids, sterols and oxygen.

Table 8.1. *Typical composition of a wort*

Constituent	Quantity ($g\ l^{-1}$)
Fructose	2.1
Glucose	9.1
Sucrose	2.3
Maltose	52.4
Maltotriose	12.8
Non-fermentable carbohydrate	23.9
Total nitrogen (as nitrogen)	0.8
Total amino acid (as nitrogen)	0.30
Total amino acid	1.65
Total phenolic constituents	0.25
Iso α acids	0.035
Calcium ions	0.065

114

Uptake of materials by yeast

Most substances of the wort diffuse freely through the yeast cell wall to the plasmalemma although some (such as hop resins, proteins and polyphenols) tend to adsorb onto the outer surface of the cell wall. Those present at the plasma membrane penetrate it readily if they are soluble in lipid, more slowly if they are water-soluble and not fat-soluble. Three methods of entry are possible, namely: simple diffusion, e.g. of undissociated organic acids; catalysed diffusion, e.g. of some sugars; and active transport, e.g. of amino acids. The first two depend on a concentration gradient but the second involves speedier entry, possibly because enzymes catalyse it. Active transport requires expenditure of energy, probably from ATP, and there is evidence that specific transport enzymes or permeases are a part of the mechanism.

Once inside the cell, not all substances are immediately used. They may survive for a short time in storage pools. Sugars are metabolised in a sequence with glucose and fructose rapidly consumed, maltose more slowly and finally maltotriose (sucrose is hydrolysed by invertase at the cell wall). Amino acids are absorbed in sequence, one group (typified by glutamate, asparagine and serine) is used before a second group (containing, for instance, histidine and leucine). Finally after an appreciable lag, amino acids in a group including glycine and tryptophan are absorbed.

Yeast metabolism

Within the cell, maltose and maltotriose are enzymatically hydrolysed to glucose. The simplest expression for fermentation is:

$$\text{Glucose} \rightarrow 2 \text{ Carbon dioxide} + 2 \text{ Ethanol} + \text{Energy.}$$
$$\text{mol wt 180} \quad 2 \times 44 \quad\quad 2 \times 46$$

This equation, named after the French scientist Gay-Lussac, shows that glucose yields almost equal weights of carbon dioxide and alcohol plus energy for the cell's activities. Unfortunately not all the energy generated can be used in a coordinated way and some escapes as heat, an important consideration in conducting large-scale fermentations.

What the equation ignores is that the yeast may be growing and also that it may be producing other metabolites, such as lactic acid, glycerol and succinic acid, albeit in relatively small quantities. Taking the question of growth into consideration, a more realistic expression of a brewery fermentation is:

$$\text{Maltose} + \text{Amino acid} \rightarrow \text{Yeast} + \text{Ethanol} + \text{Carbon dioxide} + 50 \text{ kCal Energy.}$$
$$\text{100 g} \quad\quad \text{0.5 g} \quad\quad \text{5 g} \quad \text{48.8 g} \quad\quad \text{46.8 g} \quad\quad \text{or 209 kJ}$$
$$\text{(dry weight)}$$

This contrasts markedly from the production of bakers' yeast under aerobic conditions and with sugar substrate kept low:

Sucrose + ammonia + Oxygen → Yeast + Water + Carbon dioxide + Energy.
    100 g   5 g   51 g   48 g   35 g   73 g   194 kCal
                               (dry weight)   (812 kJ)

In biochemical terms, both situations involve initially the same enzymatic pathway for the breakdown of glucose called the glycolytic or Embden–Meyerhof–Parnas (EMP) pathway (Fig. 8.1). Simplifying it, glucose is phosphorylated twice using the energy-rich ATP to produce a highly unstable molecule which splits to yield two molecules of triose phosphate. The latter will accept inorganic phosphate and is then sufficiently energy-rich not only to release ATP but to produce enol pyruvic acid phosphate, which itself releases ATP. Hence there is net output of 2 ATP for every glucose molecule used. The enol pyruvic acid is a metabolic junction. Under anaerobic conditions, it yields mainly ethanol and carbon dioxide as we have seen, but a little is converted in acetyl coenzyme A (acetyl CoA, a material important in the cell's metabolism). One of its functions is in fat and ester synthesis; another is the synthesis of amino acids.

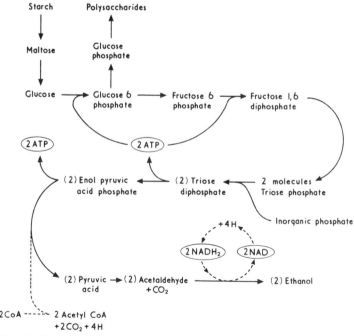

Fig. 8.1. The glycolytic (Embden–Meyerhof–Parnas) pathway for glucose dissimilation.

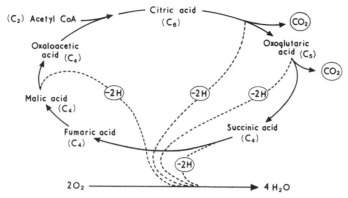

Fig. 8.2. The tricarboxylic acid, or Krebs, cycle used for aerobic metabolism of the products of the glycolytic pathway.

Figure 8.2 shows the tricarboxylic acid (TCA) cycle or Krebs cycle. In this the acetyl CoA combines with oxaloacetic acid to yield citric acid, a case of a molecule with two carbon atoms joining to one with four to give a product with six carbon atoms. By the loss of carbon dioxide, oxoglutaric acid is produced; this will combine with an ammonium ion to produce the amino acid glutamate. Alternatively an oxo-acid will react with an amino acid in such a way that the amino group is exchanged for the carbonyl group. By these amination and transamination reactions, amino acids may be synthesised.

In fully aerobic metabolism, none of the enol pyruvic acid phosphate yields ethanol. Instead the accent is on the acetyl CoA and TCA cycle. Although some amino acid synthesis will occur, preventing the completion of the cycle (as in anaerobic metabolism), most of the oxoglutaric acid produces a sequence of four-carbon organic acids until the cycle is recommenced. The significance is not the loss of two carbon dioxide molecules but the energy production. These reactions take place in the mitochondria and yield hydrogen ions which, by means of coenzymes such as nicotinamide-adenine dinucleotide (NAD), reach the terminal oxidation sites where they are oxidised by molecular oxygen. The oxidative pathway is complex and involves, among other compounds, the iron-containing cytochromes. In the oxidation, energy is released which is usefully collected by the synthesis of energy-rich coenzymes such as ATP. Respiration of 1 molecule of glucose by yeast generates 28 molecules of ATP (2 from the EMP, 2 from the TCA directly and 24 from the terminal oxidation of $NADH_2$ and a similar compound). This can be used for biosynthesis and maintenance of the cell. We know that one molecule of glucose, when chemically oxidised, provides 2.9 MJ. The 28 molecules of ATP have together an energy equivalence of only 0.854 MJ. Therefore only 29% of the total energy is harnessed; the rest escapes as heat. (Animal cells produce 38 molecules of ATP per molecule of glucose and are therefore more efficient, with 40% of the energy employed usefully.)

If a brewers' or bakers' yeast is presented with an excess of both oxygen and glucose, ethanol will be produced. This is because the mitochondria do not develop fully in the presence of glucose. Nevertheless, the mitochondria will begin to develop if the glucose concentration is reduced to a low level. This substrate inhibition, especially with glucose, is common with enzyme reactions and with entire pathways.

Aerobic metabolism is clearly more effective at yielding energy than is anaerobic metabolism. It therefore requires less glucose to meet the requirements of growth and maintenance. However if the yeast has the opportunity of metabolising ethanol aerobically, this will yield energy (for two molecules of ethanol) roughly equivalent to the difference between aerobic and anaerobic metabolism of glucose.

Not all glucose is metabolised by the EMP pathway, some goes through an entirely different route called the hexose monophosphate pathway – this yields not only energy but also pentose sugars important in the synthesis of nucleotide and nucleic acids. Some yeasts, such as *Candida utilis* (the species used for food biomass), use this pathway more effectively than does brewers' yeast and can grow on pentoses as well as hexoses.

Turning to other metabolites of yeast, if glucose is fermented under anaerobic conditions (or if acetaldehyde breakdown is blocked by adding bisulphite ions), the triose phosphate reacts with $NADH_2$ to yield glycerol. This was exploited by Germany during the 1914–18 war in the manufacture of the explosive trinitroglycerine. A similar reaction involving $NADH_2$ is possible with pyruvic acid to yield lactic acid; this happens to a small extent in yeast metabolism but assumes much more importance in muscle cells and in lactic acid bacteria. Succinic acid is also a metabolite of yeast and arises from an incomplete TCA cycle.

Production of flavour compounds

Reference has been made to oxo-acids, coenzyme A and NAD. These are known to react together enzymically in the following way:

$$RCOCOOH + \text{coenzyme A} + NAD \rightarrow RCO\,(CoA) + NADH_2 \quad + CO_2.$$
oxo-acid   + coenzyme A   acyl-CoA   + reduced NAD + carbon dioxide

The acyl CoA will then react enzymically with a variety of alcohols, for example:

$$CH_3CO\ CoA + C_2H_5OH \rightarrow CH_3COOC_2H_5 \qquad + CoA \qquad \text{, or}$$

acetyl CoA + ethanol ethyl acetate (an ester) + coenzyme A

$$C_{15}H_{31}CO\ CoA + C_3H_8O_3 \rightarrow (C_{15}H_{31}COO)_3C_3H_8 \qquad + CoA:$$

palmityl CoA + glycerol glyceryl tripalmitate (a fat) + coenzyme A

Thus esters and fats are produced. Esters are important flavour and aroma substances of beer; fats are important in the synthesis of membranes but they are substrates, just as sugars are, for the production of energy.

A variety of alcohols are produced during yeast metabolism and have some influence on beer flavour. They are derived from oxo-acids which are produced either from carbohydrate metabolism (e.g. pyruvic acid or oxoglutaric acid) or from amino acids by transamination with an existing oxo-acid (Fig. 8.3). From oxovalerate, it is possible to aminate or transaminate enzymically to yield valine. Alternatively, oxovalerate will enzymically decarboxylate to produce isobutyraldehyde which will then reduce, by means of $NADH_2$ and alcohol dehydrogenase, to give isobutanol. This is analogous to pyruvate giving ethanol and carbon dioxide.

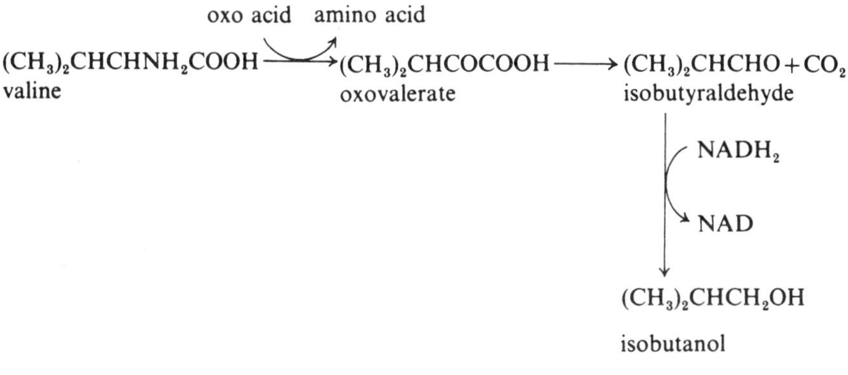

oxo acid   amino acid

$(CH_3)_2CHCHNH_2COOH \longrightarrow (CH_3)_2CHCOCOOH \longrightarrow (CH_3)_2CHCHO + CO_2$

valine   oxovalerate   isobutyraldehyde

$NADH_2$

NAD

$(CH_3)_2CHCH_2OH$

isobutanol

A wide range of alcohols are produced in this way, not only aliphatic ones but also the aromatic phenylethanol.

Diketones such as diacetyl are powerful flavour substances. In yeast they arise from the excretion of the compound acetolactate

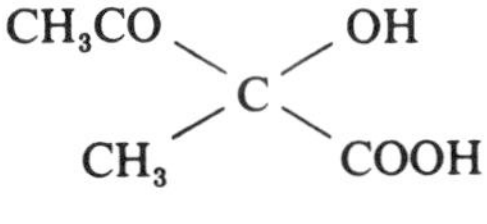

CH_3CO , OH
      $>C<$ into the medium. It decarboxylates and
CH_3 , $COOH$

oxidises chemically (not enzymically) in the fermenting wort or beer to give diacetyl ($CH_3COCOCH_3$). Yeast is capable of reducing diacetyl as

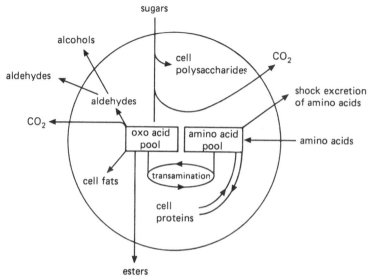

Fig. 8.3. The origin of fusel alcohols, esters and aldehydes in the yeast cell.

it diffuses back into the cell by a reductase enzyme and $NADH_2$ to produce 2,3 butanediol ($CH_3CHOHCHOHCH_3$), which is almost flavourless. Diacetyl however gives a strong butterscotch taste and aroma in beer at 1 ppm.

Sulphur compounds are potent flavour and aroma substances. They arise primarily from organic sulphur compounds in wort, such as the amino acid methionine or sulphur-containing proteins. Alternatively, in the absence of organic sources of sulphur, flavour compounds arise from sulphate ions. Hydrogen sulphide is the simplest of the sulphur volatiles and is produced particularly during active yeast growth. Another simple compound is dimethyl sulphide ($CH_3)_2S$ which arises from the compound S-methylmethionine present in malt and wort. The flavour thresholds for hydrogen sulphide and dimethyl sulphide are 10–30 and 20–30 ppb respectively.

Top and bottom cropping yeasts

Early in the nineteenth century, most countries practising brewing were using yeasts which rose to the surface of the fermenting wort towards the end of fermentation and could be skimmed away for reuse. Many of these yeasts were inefficient in fermentation and therefore the more progressive brewers were interested at least in experimenting with the yeasts used in Munich, which had better fermentative powers. These were strains that sank to the base of the fermentor towards the end of the fermentation. From 1842 onwards, the Munich strains were adopted with spectacular success in Czechoslovakia, Denmark and the USA. By the turn of the century, the Carlsberg brewery in Copenhagen had developed methods of isolating single cells of yeast and growing up a clone of pure culture sufficient to inoculate fermentors of commercial scale. This also helped to spread bottom yeasts to all countries that wished to share the new brewing technology.

Britain and to a lesser extent Belgium, Canada and the Cologne area of Germany had very satisfactory top yeasts and continue to use them. Nevertheless, bottom yeasts now dominate in Belgium and Canada; this is also true of Scotland. The differences between top and bottom yeasts, quite apart from the more hydrophobic surface of the top yeasts, relate mainly to temperature of fermentation, beer flavour and aroma. Top yeasts are commonly operated in the range 15–22 °C, bottom yeasts in the range 8–15 °C. At the higher temperature, top yeast fermentation is faster. The differences in flavour and aroma relate partly to the yeast and partly to the fermentation temperature. Some UK breweries produce their 'lagers' with top yeasts, but often at lower temperatures.

With the development of large fermentors, especially those of cylindroconical shape, the distinction between top and bottom yeasts tends to disappear. Top yeasts can be encouraged at the end of fermentation to accumulate in the cone and this is convenient from the standpoint of separating them cleanly from the beer above. Nevertheless, ales are usually produced in these vessels by top yeasts and lagers, at lower temperatures, by bottom yeasts.

Course of batch fermentation

The products of fermentation are ethanol, carbon dioxide and energy (including heat). Carbon dioxide produced in very substantial weights is extremely dangerous; about 4% of this gas in air by volume can cause asphyxiation in a short time and levels in breweries may well be limited to 0.5% in the future. Enclosed vessels are, therefore, safer (except for those who enter them). It is possible to collect the carbon dioxide from enclosed vessels and use it in post-fermentation processes, but only after expensive equipment has been used to purify and compress it. With open vessels, it is necessary to have very efficient air flow through fermentation halls in order to disperse the gas. Carbon dioxide is extremely dense and therefore tends to accumulate at floor level or below floors. Evolution of carbon dioxide also has the tendency to cause a small loss of ethanol.

Heat evolution during fermentation is equivalent to about 0.6 MJ kg^{-1} of glucose equivalent or 3.5 kJ l^{-1} h^{-1}. In order to maintain a selected fermentation temperature, it is necessary to have cooling devices in or on fermentors. These may take the form of copper or stainless steel tubular coils within the vessels or hollow jackets on the walls. The coolant may be water, brine or a simple alcohol. Vessels are usually stainless steel but a small number or copper or copper-lined vessels still survive.

The aerated wort arriving from the coolers is not absolutely sterile. Small numbers of wort bacteria present are capable of multiplying quickly unless fermentation by yeast is encouraged so that the pH of the wort falls and ethanol is produced. The yeast slurry itself is a potential reservoir of bacteria that survive fermentation and, as far as possible, this contamination should be avoided.

It is imperative that the yeast be active, with over 85% of the cells viable, as measured by the cells resisting staining with methylene blue dye in a buffer solution of pH 5. The important consideration is that the yeast grows and ferments after the shortest possible lag phase. Inoculation rates are high in commercial brewing (1.5–2.5 g pressed weight per litre). This represents 20–25% of the yeast cropped from a batch of fermented wort equal in volume to the one to be inoculated. Such an inoculum therefore only multiplies 4–5-fold, equivalent to each cell dividing by budding 2–3 times.

Ale fermentation using a top yeast is conducted with an initial wort temperature of 15–16 °C but this value is allowed to rise slowly, controlled by cooling coils or jackets, until (typically) at 36 h it has reached 20–25 °C. Activity is evident from the accumulation of yeasty foam on the surface and also from carbon dioxide evolution. Cooling is then gradually increased to bring the temperature down to about 17 °C at 72 h (Fig. 8.4). Little fermentation occurs over the last 10 h and the yeast will tend to rise to the surface in traditional fermentors. It is

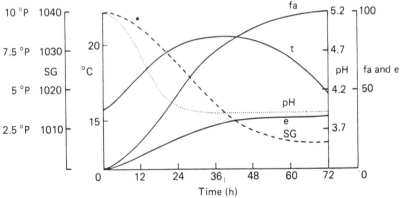

Fig. 8.4. The course of a top fermentation with an ale yeast. SG, specific gravity of the wort; t, temperature; Fa, fusel alcohol content (in mg l^{-1}); e, ester content (in mg l^{-1}).

skimmed mechanically or sucked off from the surface and stored at low temperature before being filtered to recover entrapped beer (or 'barm ale' as it is called). Typically, a wort of SG 1.040 (10 °P) is fermented to 1.008–1.010 (2–2.5 °P).

The equipment used for ale fermentation was traditionally an open vessel, either square or round in plan, of wooden construction with 50–200 hl capacity and with a depth of 2–4 m. More modern ale fermentors are of stainless steel construction and, to aid automatic 'cleaning in place', they tend to be enclosed. Their capacity is usually in the range 150–500 hl. In plan view they are rectangular and the wort depth is usually 3–5 m.

In Britain, the fermentor is often used as the gauging vessel for Customs and Excise and a reference dip plate is fitted to the lip of the vessel. From here the distance is measured to the surface of the wort; from previous calibrations on the particular vessel, the volume of wort can be computed. Excise is paid on this volume multiplied by the wort strength – say 10 °P, not on the alcoholic strength of the final beer.

Lager fermentations were traditionally carried out in open vessels but almost all lager is now produced in enclosed vessels, either like the modern ale fermentors or alternatively in cylindroconical fermentors or other vessels of large capacity. The aerated wort arrives at the fermentor at 7–11 °C. Like the ale wort, it is inoculated with yeast either in the pipes leading to the fermentor or within the vessel itself. Because of the lower temperature, fermentation is slower than it is for ale production. A traditional bottom fermentation takes 8–10 days. It begins with a slow rise in temperature of the wort, carefully checked by the use of the cooling coils or jackets, up to a maximum of 10–15 °C. This takes some 3–5 days. Activity is indicated by the accumulation of

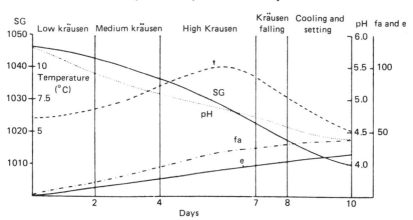

Fig. 8.5. The course of a traditional bottom fermentation with a lager yeast. SG, specific gravity of the wort; t, temperature; fa, fusel alcohol content (in mg l^{-1}); e, ester content (in mg l^{-1}).

a yeasty foam on the wort surface and evolution of carbon dioxide. The foam can become similar to cauliflower heads and is referred to as 'Krausen' or curls. For the rest of the fermentation, the temperature is reduced by use of the cooling elements. The Krausen falls and the yeast begins to accumulate at the base of the vessel (Fig. 8.5). For traditional lagering, the brewer retains some fermentable sugar in the beer. Thus, for a lager wort of SG 1.044 (11 °P), the primary fermentation will bring this value to about SG 1.011. For what is called the ageing process, the wort is completely fermented out.

Continuous fermentation

Patented methods of continuous fermentation of wort have existed for some 80 years. Had modern materials, methods of construction, and sterilisation techniques been available, several of them would have been feasible. Two methods of continuous fermentation were introduced successfully between 1959 and 1962. One comprises a series of stirred tanks (Fig. 8.6) into the first of which is introduced yeast and a continuous stream of wort. The wort is fermented by the yeast and overflows into a succeeding vessel. The degree to which it is fermented is a function of (i) the temperature, (ii) the dwell-time of the wort in the vessel and (iii) the strength of the wort. With fully mixed vessel contents where the yeast is inoculated once, an equilibrium becomes established in each vessel in a chain of fermentors. With a wort of SG 1.040, the outflow from the first vessel might be 1.020 and the yeast population (say 30×10^6 cells ml^{-1}), and from the second vessel 1.010 and 40×10^6 respectively. This specific gravity and yeast count are determined by the wort flow-rate, the temperature and the wort strength. If there is a constant recycling of yeast into the first vessel, this will greatly influence fermentation so that a higher relative flow-rate of wort may be employed to achieve the same equilibrium values. In practice, the total dwell-time of wort in the entire multi-vessel system was 24–30 h.

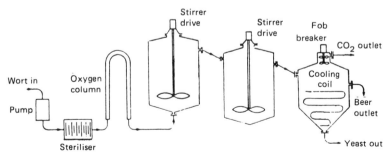

Fig. 8.6. A system of continuous fermentation using two stirred vessels in cascade. A fob breaker is a device used to prevent accumulation of foam.

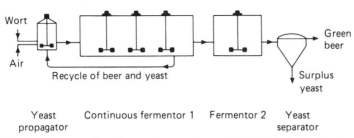

Fig. 8.7. A system of continuous fermentation used in New Zealand with three stirred vessels in cascade and yeast recycling.

Such cascade fermentors (Fig. 8.7) were (until very recently) used to produce almost all New Zealand beer. In the UK they were employed in some four or five breweries but have now virtually been abandoned. They proved expensive compared with modern batch vessels in both capital and revenue costs. One suffered from an infection from a wild yeast that secreted a zymocide. The zymocide operating in constant conditions at its optimum pH value killed all the culture yeast and the wild yeast dominated the system. There were also problems associated with high levels of yeast growth in some instances.

A second type of continuous fermentor comprises a vertical cylindrical vessel or tower into the bottom of which sterile wort is pumped (Fig. 8.8). The vessel is inoculated with a strongly sedimenting yeast but, at the base of the vessel, the aggregations of the yeast are deflocculated by the high concentration of wort sugars. Although some mixing of the contents of the vessel occurs, there is substantial plug flow up the vessel. Thus the contents at a height of 3 m from the bottom of the vessel might be said, for instance, to be like that of a batch fermentation 24 h old; those 6 m from the bottom like a 2 day old batch fermentation, etc. Wort flow is so adjusted that when the fermenting wort reaches the top of the vessel, it is fermented to the required degree. As the fermentation progresses, the yeast reacquires its flocculent properties and therefore tends to sediment against the upward flow of wort. At the top of the vessel is a decanting device which provides an inclined surface to further encourage separation of yeast, allowing beer substantially free of yeast to flow on to post-fermentation treatments.

A typical tower was some 8 m to the decanter and 9 m overall in height and its diameter about 2 m. With a total working capacity of 65 hl, hourly rates of beer production of 16.5 hl are achievable. This is equivalent to a dwell-time of 4 h, but something double that dwell-time was normally needed to get a beer which matched reasonably with its batch equivalent. The average amount of pressed yeast produced was 1.1 kg hl^{-1}, very much like a batch process. At one time, something

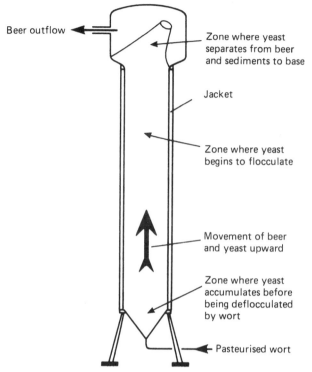

Beer outflow

Zone where yeast
separates from beer
and sediments to base

Jacket

Zone where yeast
begins to flocculate

Movement of beer
and yeast upward

Zone where yeast
accumulates before
being deflocculated
by wort

Pasteurised wort

Fig. 8.8. A system of continuous fermentation using a tower reactor and a highly sedimentary yeast.

approaching 4% of British beer was produced by the tower continuous fermentors. However flavour matching with batch beers was often difficult, especially with lagers. There were infection problems, particularly with lactic acid bacteria and there was a difficult period of 2–3 weeks from start-up until something approaching equilibrium was achieved. It was possible to run a fermentor for 6–9 months without cleaning but the capital and revenue costs were high compared with modern batch systems. Because of these costs, the problems of flavour matching, of start-up and infection, the tower system has now been virtually abandoned except for vinegar production.

Modern developments in fermentor design

Large enclosed batch vessels are not new. Before 1960, there were stainless steel vessels of 11 500 hl capacity, but such vessels were not designed for automatic 'cleaning in place' (CIP). Since that time, stainless steel vessels have been designed and built with the following design features: (i) automatic CIP systems, (ii) self-generating mixing

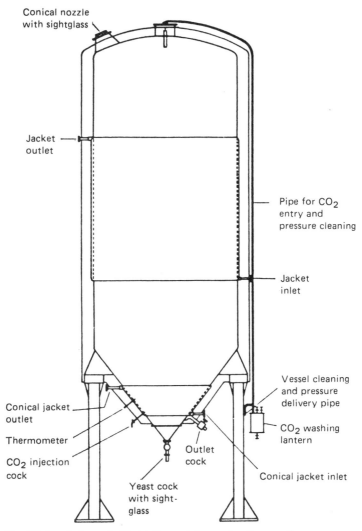

Fig. 8.9. A cylindroconical batch fermentation maturation vessel.

currents, (iii) temperature control with cooling jackets, (iv) bases that encourage yeast sedimentation, and (v) carbon dioxide collection. Probably the most successful have been the cylindroconical fermentors which range in size from 100–4800 hl. They have a sharp cone with an included angle of 60–75° (Fig. 8.9), a height of up to 20 m and a diameter of up to 10.5 m. Usually they are constructed of cold-rolled stainless steel, which has a surface which is particularly easy to clean.

Not all large vessels are of the cylindroconical shape; some are squat cylinders (7.5 m diameter and 12 m height) with a gently sloping base.

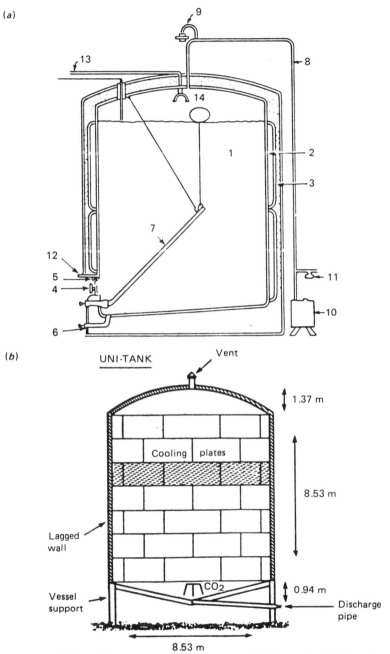

Fig. 8.10 *a*. Large outdoor fermentation vessel (USP 3, 374, 726). 1. Tank;
2. Cooling jacket; 3. Foamed-synthetic resin; 4. Manhole; 5. Beer drainage cock;
6. Beer feed pipe; 7. Beer discharge pipe (pivoted); 8. Exhaust pipe; 9. Siphon
breaker; 10. Pressure relief valve; 11. Vacuum breaker; 12. Thermometer and
liquid depth senser; 13. Water and detergent supply pipe; 14. Water and
detergent spray. *b*. The Unitank, a batch fermentor or maturation vessel.

These cannot be cooled easily by wall jackets and therefore the contents are pumped through a pipework loop incorporating a plate heat exchanger chiller. Still other vessels are between the two extremes with a blunt cone having a 155° included angle, a diameter of 8.5 m and a height of 9 m (Fig. 8.10).

The rationale for large vessels is that their cost is only 30–37% greater than those half their size. The cost ratio is said to be close to the volume ratio raised to the power of 0.65. Nevertheless, there are difficulties. Surfaces of vessels are small compared with their volume. Cooling may therefore be slow – say 0.5 °C h^{-1}, or even less. Strong cooling with jackets may lead to ice forming close to the jackets on the inside of the vessel while the average fermenting wort temperature is 10 °C. Another problem is that the vessel may accommodate several batches of wort some of which will be inoculated with yeast, but usually not all. Filling is thus slow – as is emptying. A very large volume is at stake and such a volume can only be feasible if the brewery has one or more brands of beer selling at appropriately high volumes. Yet large volumes of liquid are not readily influenced by ambient temperatures so that these fermentors are often sited outside in tank farms, subject to perhaps tropical heat or arctic cold.

With very tall vessels, strong circulatory currents develop during fermentation. Evolution of a bubble of carbon dioxide at the base of the vessel where hydrostatic pressure is high is followed by a rapid rise of as much as 20 m to the surface. This encourages upward flow of fermenting wort except near the vessel perimeter where flow tends to be downwards, helped by the action of the cooling jackets. The strong circulatory currents speed up fermentation and therefore ale fermentations are usually completed in 3 days or less and lager fermentations in 3–6 days, depending on the temperature.

At the end of the fermentation, it is advantageous to bring the yeast (top or bottom strain) into the cone. It is kept cold by a cone jacket. Under ideal circumstances, the yeast can be run off with a relatively small volume of beer and transferred to awaiting fermentors as the inoculum for new fermentations. The beer, on the other hand, will have little entrained yeast. In practice, many yeasts do not separate from the beer so precisely and require centrifugal separation. Where discrete separation can be achieved, it is possible to carry out post-fermentation treatment of the beer without moving it to another vessel. This is desirable in that the picking up of dissolved oxygen during transfer is avoided. Such oxygen causes problems of chill-haze and flavour instability in packaged beer.

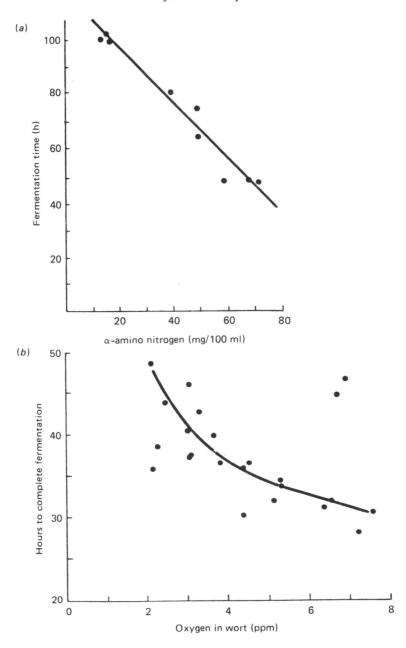

(a)

Fermentation time (h)

α-amino nitrogen (mg/100 ml)

(b)

Hours to complete fermentation

Oxygen in wort (ppm)

Control of fermentation

With traditional batch fermentation, some control can be exercised with respect to speed of fermentation by the wort temperature and the size of the yeast inoculum. To a lesser extent, it is possible to encourage faster fermentations by stirring.

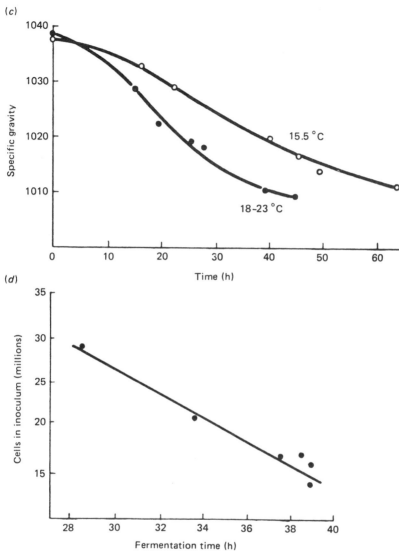

Fig. 8.11. Relationship of fermentation parameters in a cylindroconical batch fermentation between fermentation time and (*a*) wort α amino acid content; (*b*) dissolved oxygen content of the wort, (*c*) temperature and (*d*) number of yeast cells inoculated (10^6 ml^{-1}).

More control is possible with respect to modern batch fermentors. Temperature and yeast concentration are again controlled (Fig. 8.11) but there is, in addition, a greater possibility of control through the dissolved-oxygen content of the wort and the amino acids content of the wort. This has led to strict specifications on these last two parameters. In many cases, the levels of both have been reduced, not with a primary view of slowing fermentation but instead of restricting yeast growth. This is because wort carbohydrate used in yeast growth is lost to ethanol production. A brewer gets a poor financial return for his surplus yeast compared with that for his beer.

Mention has been made in earlier chapters of high-gravity brewing. In cylindroconical fermentors the fermentation time is increased only by 20–25% for a 50% increase of wort strength. There is therefore great advantage in high-gravity brewing from the standpoint of vessel utilisation, quite apart from the advantages in wort boiling and cooling.

Some beers, called light or lite beers, have virtually all the wort carbohydrate fermented instead of some 70–80%. This is achieved in most cases by adding fungal amyloglucosidase to the fermenting wort. The dextrins are degraded to fermentable glucose by the enzyme during the course of the fermentation. Final SG values may be 1.000 or lower. In practice, this procedure adds a further day to the fermentation time. A spin-off is that beer of this kind is ideal for packaged shandies. With an ethanol content of say 4.5% v/v, the beer will be mixed with as much as 9 volumes of lemonade or ginger ale. This gives a final ethanol content of say 0.45% v/v (which is considered to be non-alcoholic for trade and legal purposes).

Other fermentations

Wine and cider may be fermented by the microorganisms found naturally on grapes and apples. There is less control of quality than when the juice is sterilised or strongly treated with sulphur dioxide (up to 200 ppm). Yeast cultures are then specially selected to grow well in the presence of sulphur dioxide and to produce excellent flavours and aromas. They are strains of the yeast *Saccharomyces cerevisiae* var. *ellipsoideus*. Many wine-producing countries including Australia, Germany, USA and South Africa use specially selected and propagated yeast cultures. The same applies to the major cider producers. Scrumpy is the farmhouse cider produced using the natural flora on the apples.

In white wine production, comparatively low temperatures (10–15 °C) are maintained and the fermentation extends for 2 weeks or more. The temperature is usually in the range 20–30 °C for red wine fermentations. Suspended in the juice (or must) are skins, seeds and stalks. Rosé wines are produced by very early removal of these solids; red wines which are to be drunk soon after production (e.g. Beaujolais Nouveau) also have the solids removed early in the fermentation. Red wines, rich in colour (and therefore tannins), are in contact with this pomace for much of the fermentation. Ethanol contents of wine range from 8 to 13% v/v.

Sulphur dioxide not only prevents microbial infection of the must, it

Table 8.2. *The basis of beverages with alcoholic strengths over 20% by volume*

Raw material	Treatment	Product
Barley ⟶ Mash or wash fermented, distilled		Irish whiskey
Barley malt ⟶ Mash or wash fermented, distilled		Scotch malt whisky, Scotch grain whisky
Maize ⟶ Mash or wash fermented, distilled		Potable alcohol (for vodka and gin)
Rice	Mash or wash fermented, not distilled	Sake
Molasses	Fermented and distilled	Rum
Apples	Fermented to give cider, distilled to give	Calvados, applejack
Grapes	Fermented to give wine, distilled to give	Brandy, marc

also aids separation of the must from the pomace and prevents browning of white wines. The best juice is that which separates easily from the pomace, the free-running must. That which requires pressing to recover it from the pomace is used for inferior wines, which are often distilled. Brandy (Table 8.2) is derived from the best wine by distillation while cruder distillation of the poorer wines yields marc, which is richer in products other than ethanol (the so-called fuel oils).

Fortified wines are those to which ethanol (pure or as brandy) has been added. The simplest to understand is port which is produced by arresting fermentation by the addition of alcohol. Sherry involves a complex secondary fermentation with a second yeast before fortification. Madeira achieves some of its characteristic flavour from heating the wine – Californian sherry has similarities in processing and in flavour. In the middle of the nineteenth century, most burgundies imported into Britain had 14–16% ethanol. They had been fortified (or in more picturesque language subjected to *le travail à l'anglaise*).

Sparkling wines are produced either by a secondary fermentation in bottle (e.g. Champagne) or in tank (e.g. Sparkling Saumur) or by direct carbonation of wine in tank (e.g. the cheapest of the Spanish Champañ). The yeast is removed from bottles of Champagne by encouraging it into the neck of the bottle, freezing the neck and discharging the yeast as a solid plug. Wine and brandy mixture are added to make up the volume.

Turning to distilled beverages other than brandy, whisky is made by fermenting a malt mash (or malt and adjunct mash) with *Saccharomyces cerevisiae* strains (Table 8.2). Often a mixture of brewing yeast and specially propagated distilling yeast is used. The fermented mash (or wash as it is called) is distilled so that the yeast is killed. Gin is made from potable alcohol produced in a similar way. In gin distillation, fusel oil is not permitted in the final product. The potable alcohol is redistilled in such a way that the vapours pass through 'botanicals' comprising juniper berries, angelica, lemon peel, coriander, orris, cinnamon and liquorice. Vodka is also grain-based and is not only carefully subjected to a stringently selective distillation, like gin and whisky, but to filtration through activated carbon. Rum is a product of fermenting molasses and then distilling; white rum is treated, like vodka, to carbon filtration.

Yeast products

Some yeast surplus to the British brewers' requirements is sent to the Scottish distilleries. A further use is in yeast extracts, particularly for pharmaceutical purposes or for the flavour of food. The hop bitter substances are removed from the yeast by dilute alkali before autolysis (self-digestion) of the cells. In the autolytic procedure for pharmaceutical tablets, the cells are held at 45 °C for 12–24 h in the presence of small volumes of chloroform or ethyl acetate. The extract is clarified and concentrated to a syrup or spray-dried. For flavouring extracts, the yeast is mixed with a high concentration of salts, sugar or certain acetate esters to form a slurry. The low molecular weight materials are extracted in the process and are concentrated to give a salty meat-flavoured material. This is rich in amino acids, vitamins and nucleotides.

Yeast is also a source of the enzyme invertase (which is secreted by the cells to hydrolyse sucrose). Dried yeast preparations can be produced that are rich in the enzyme. They are used either for sucrose inversion or, more interestingly, in the making of soft-centred chocolates. The filler of the centres starts off as a solid mix of sucrose granules, yeast preparation and flavouring. It is coated with chocolate before the invertase hydrolyses the sucrose and thus liquefies the filling.

9   Post-fermentation treatments

Beer run off from the fermentor is not ready for drinking. It requires a variety of treatments before it is despatched from the brewery. Six processes are involved, namely:

(a)   carbonation,
(b)   flavour and aroma modification,
(c)   colour standardising,
(d)   stabilisation against non-biological haze and flavour change,
(e)   clarification, and
(f)   biological stabilisation.

Traditional cask ale

The processes do not necessarily follow in the above sequence. The simplest series of treatments relates to traditional cask ale. Here the beer is run from fermentor to a long shallow vessel called a racking back which is usually enclosed (Fig. 9.1). From the racking back are flexible pipes for filling the individual casks. With an enclosed back, it is possible to speed beer flow by pressurising it. That also gives the opportunity of counterpressuring each cask by having a seal at the point where the fill pipe enters and providing a return pipe to the back

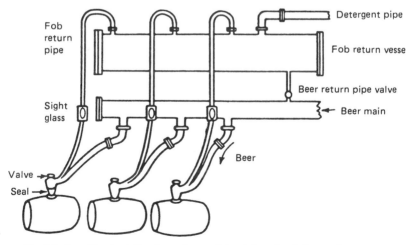

Fig. 9.1. A racking back for dispensing traditional draught ale into casks.

or another vessel. Air from the cask, displaced by the beer, is thus carried away along with foam and excess beer. The counterpressuring also helps to keep the carbon dioxide in solution in the beer.

The beer should have active yeast cells in suspension to a concentration of about $0.25\text{--}2.00 \times 10^6$ cells ml^{-1}. Another requirement is fermentable sugar, either present in the beer but more often added as syrup called 'primings'. Some 0.35–2.00 l are added for each hectolitre of beer, either to the racking back or directly to the cask. The syrup has an SG of 1.150 and comprises cane or beet sugar plus maltose-rich starch hydrolysate plus caramel. It provides (i) a fermentable substrate for secondary fermentation in the cask, (ii) sweetening, and (iii) colouring.

Secondary fermentation proceeds in the cask and provides, when the cask is bunged (sealed) with a wooden peg, additional carbonation that is necessary if primary fermentation took place in a shallow open vessel. Other additions are made to the cask before it is bunged. In order to bring the yeast out of suspension and into the belly of the cask, isinglass finings are added; these are described later. Hop material is often added, either as hop cones, pellets or as essential oil. This contributes nothing to bitterness but does give the beer a distinctive hoppy aroma because of the essential oils. A further addition may be sodium metabisulphite to provide the bacteriostatic sulphur dioxide at a maximum level of 70 ppm, but more usually 20–5 ppm.

After a period of secondary fermentation, the impervious wooden peg in the cask may be replaced by a permeable one (that is, with the xylem vessels in the wood running along rather than across the peg). This permits excess carbon dioxide to escape. When the cask has been delivered, wedged into position on its belly, it can be broached by driving a tap assembly into a wooden bung set on the end (or head) of the cask. The bung flies into the beer and the tap wedges firmly into position in the keystone ring which surrounded the bung.

Cask beer is relatively inexpensive to process because it requires relatively little energy to produce. Its production is, however, labour-intensive and casks (even the modern aluminium ones) are difficult to clean. It also uses a lot of floor space, largely because of storing and cleaning casks.

Isinglass finings

The finings – employed in clarifying beer – are the most curious material used in brewing. They are derived from the swim-bladders of tropical fishes, that is the organ that enables a fish to maintain its depth in water. The organ in the large tropical fishes is substantial and even when dried weighs several hundred grams. It is almost pure collagen and therefore has long polypeptide chains, three coiling around each other to form the protein molecule. The individual chains are given frequent sharp coiling twists due to the presence of adjacent imino acids, proline and hydroxyproline; they are held together principally by hydrogen bonding. They have an overall positive charge but limited regions may carry negative charges.

Brewery finings are manufactured by slicing the swim-bladders and soaking them in cold dilute acid for several weeks. This produces a turbid colourless viscous solution which is only stable when kept cold. Finings quickly denature at ambient temperatures to yield gelatin that has little value. In this connection, many USA breweries use gelatin but this is manufactured by alkaline degradation of mammalian collagen. Its clarifying properties are less pronounced than isinglass finings.

The finings are effective because the long molecules fall through the beer like a net, greatly aided by the electrical charges. They associate strongly with the negatively charged yeast cells and yet may protrude from the cells to enmesh further cells. Additionally the finings associate with other charged material in the beer, notably proteins and lipids. The coagulum that forms settles in 1–4 h. Vigorous shaking, as when the cask is rolled, partly disperses the coagulated lees but a good sample of finings will reclarify the beer several times.

Some beers fail to clarify adequately with isinglass-finings treatment because of excessive quantities of positively charged material in suspension. Such beers may be pretreated with what is called auxiliary finings, usually based on alginates and negatively charged. Overtreatment with auxiliary finings means that expensive isinglass finings are used to neutralise the excess, before the isinglass can be effective in clarifying. With yeast cells in the range $0.25–2.5 \times 10^6$ cells ml^{-1}, it is usual for isinglass finings to be added at 1% by volume to beer.

Secondary fermentation in tank

There is a difficulty in nomenclature because no clear definitions have been agreed, but (in most cases) lagering, maturation, conditioning and ruh treatment mean almost the same. In traditional processing, beer from the open primary fermentor was run into an enclosed lager tank. It had to have a count of active yeast of $2–5 \times 10^6$ cells ml^{-1} and also an adequate level of fermentable sugars (1–1.5 °P).

These requirements were met by some yeasts of very moderate sedimenting ability but, with very flocculent strains, too little yeast was left in suspension and too much fermentable matter. With very non-flocculent strains, too much yeast was present in suspension and these cells had virtually fermented out all the wort sugars. There were three solutions to the dilemma. A brewery could operate with a flocculent strain using half the fermentors and a quite separate, non-flocculent strain fermenting in the remaining vessels. The lagering tanks were filled with a mixture of the two kinds of beer, one providing fermentable sugar and the other active yeast. Alternatively fermenting wort at the Krausen stage would be run into a lagering tank as 5–10% of the contents and, when mixed with fermented beer from the primary fermentors, would provide both the fermentable sugars and the active yeast. Finally, a non-flocculent yeast could be largely, but not completely, removed from beer (ex-primary fermentor) by means of a centrifuge at a stage when fermentable sugar was still present.

Assuming that secondary fermentation has started in the lager tank, carbon dioxide is at first permitted to escape. It carries with it from the tank several unwanted volatiles such as oxygen and hydrogen sulphide. After this purging, the tank is completely closed so that beer becomes carbonated. The temperature is then brought down, by cooling coils or jackets, to 0 °C. Yeast tends to settle along with other suspended matter. There is one school of thought that believes that complex chemical changes take place as the beer is held for 2–4 weeks at low temperature. Another says that the only important consideration is the levels of the diketone diacetyl and of dissolved oxygen. Certainly it is imperative to reduce dissolved oxygen levels to 0.2 ppm or below.

There has been considerable economic pressure to reduce lagering time. It can cost about £0.06 day^{-1} hl^{-1}. This has led to the development of several new techniques. In the USA, many breweries practise the ageing process. Apart from one major US company, this means fermenting beer to completion in primary fermentation, making sure that there is no dissolved oxygen and little diacetyl in the beer, and then holding the beer at 2–4 °C for 2–4 days. Another process involves a 'diacetyl rest' immediately after primary fermentation at a temperature of 12–18 °C for about a week, followed by a week's cold lagering. The diacetyl rest gives optimum conditions for the yeast to release all the acetolactate that is possible and additionally to reduce it enzymically the diacetyl (see Chapter 7). This is similar to the old UK system of warm conditioning followed by cold conditioning. The least expensive treatment (but probably not the best) is to chill the beer from the primary fermentor and to carbonate it artificially.

Additions to the lagering tank

The lagering or conditioning tank is a convenient place for various additives related to (i) adjusting flavour, aroma and colour, (ii) bacteriostasis, (iii) enhancement of foaming ability and (iv) stabilising beer against flavour deterioration and haze formation in packaged beer.

Bitterness can be increased by the addition of isomerised hop extract, in other words iso α acid. This has to be well mixed and care must be taken to ensure that it dissolves. Hop-oil preparations may be added to increase hoppy aroma either in the form of distillate of hops or a carbon dioxide extract rich in essential oils. Some ales receive sweetening in the conditioning tank by the addition of priming sugars; this may adjust beer colour. Alternatively colour may be adjusted by addition of caramel.

Bacteriostasis in some countries, such as the UK, may only be achieved by addition of sulphur dioxide or producers of it. In some other countries it may be possible to add other materials such as octyl gallate (3,4,5-trihydroxybenzoic acid). Agents which may be used effectively to increase the ability of beer to foam include alginate esters of cellulose derivatives, various gums and saponin. Their action will be discussed in the next section, as will flavour and haze stabilisation.

Beer foaming

It is thought that when beer discharges bubbles of carbon dioxide, the foam produced is partly stabilised by a migration of substances of hydrophobic character to the bubble surface or gas/liquid interface. These will include glycoproteins with molecules comprising a hydrophobic protein head and a long hydrophilic carbohydrate tail. The heads stabilise the bubble surface while the tails give local high viscosity to the beer between the bubbles and this hinders drainage of beer from the foam (Fig. 9.2).

Other hydrophobic molecules will compete with the protein for

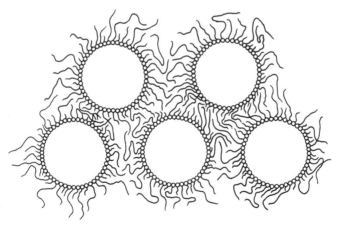

Fig. 9.2. The structure of beer foam. The bubbles attract to their surface a variety of molecules with hydrophobic heads. Some have long hydrophilic tails that increase local viscosity and impede the drainage of beer from the foam.

positions on the bubble surfaces and may detract from the foaming; these include essential oils and lipids. If, however, the lipid was attached to carbohydrate, it might be a foam-positive molecule (i.e., might enhance beer foam). Substances that enhance foaming include hop resins, dextrins, β glucans and melanoidins, presumably because they cause local high viscosity or may chemically associate with substances at the bubble surfaces. The most effective foam enhancers will have not only these properties but will also cross-link with the glycoproteins to rigidify the bubble wall (e.g. the alginate esters). Another point is that the hydrophobic material is virtually at the limit of its solubility; this is excellent, providing that the foaming occurs in the customer's glass and not in the beer being processed.

The bubbles need to be of similar small size because large bubbles will capture small ones and this tears a foam apart. Another point is that carbon dioxide readily dissolves in liquid and its foam is relatively unstable compared with air or nitrogen foams. Some beers therefore have air or nitrogen introduced into them as the beverages are dispensed into the customer's glass.

Beer haze

Hazes may arise because of the presence of microorganisms in the beer and these are normally removed by filtration. With respect to non-biological hazes, it is possible to have problems arising from suspensions of calcium oxalate or from β glucan gums. Nevertheless the majority of hazes that arise after packaging are due to protein–tannin complexes coming out of solution.

During wort boiling, wort cooling and subsequent beer chilling, protein associated or tanned by polyphenol comes out of solution as 'trub'. Beer at the beginning of lagering will, if chilled to 0 °C throw what is called a 'chill haze'. Such a haze will normally disappear when the beer is warmed. But beer held in package for a long time will produce a haze stable at ambient temperature, the so-called permanent haze. It will disappear only when the beer is heated to about 70 °C and will reappear as the temperature falls.

When analysed, the protein precursor of chill or permanent haze can be shown to be a mixture of small proteins or polypeptides with a range of molecular weights 10000–60000 and with isoelectric points between pH 3 and 5.5. This contrasts with the proteins associated with beer foam, which have molecular weights (according to gel filtration) of 10000–15000, isoelectric points between pH 5.5 and 8.0 and are associated with massive amounts of carbohydrate. There may be in these hazes up to 25% carbohydrate associated with haze protein but this pales against the 75–85% commonly encountered with foam

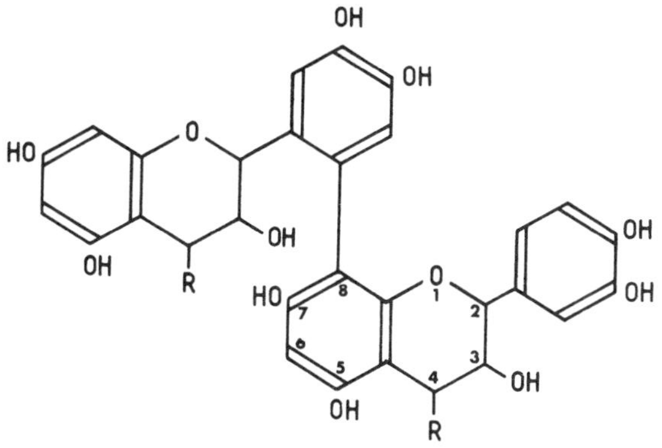

Fig. 9.3. Structure of a proanthocyanin or anthocyanogen that is likely to be important in beer haze production. It is a dimer of a polyphenol.

protein. Both types arise principally from the barley storage protein, hordein.

The polyphenol material that appears to react particularly actively with the protein is thought to be the dimers and trimers of certain proanthocyanins or anthocyanogens (Fig. 9.3). There are several hypotheses as to how the reaction takes place; one suggests that the polyphenol becomes activated in the presence of dissolved oxygen and a heavy metal ion catalyst, such as iron or copper. The activated molecule then combines with one, possibly more than one, molecule of protein. This in turn attracts further molecules of polyphenol and protein to it. At some stage, this mass built from the 'bricks' of protein and tannin will exceed its solubility and come out of solution.

To combat the possibility of haze developing in packaged beer, it is clear that dissolved oxygen and heavy metal ions must be avoided. Particularly serious metals in this respect are tin, titanium and lead. Good practice will ensure low dissolved oxygen levels (0.2 ppm or below) but methods of reducing them include additions of reducing agents such as sodium metabisulphite and ascorbic acid to the beer.

One of the best methods of combating haze is to chill the beer to as low a temperature as possible before the final filtration. By this means, a great deal of the protein–tannin complex that acts as haze precursor will come out of solution and be filtered. Another approach is to balance protein and polyphenol as nearly as can be achieved. Thus a beer with excess protein and insufficient polyphenol will have tannic acid added. Protein is then precipitated. Alternatively, the protein may be treated with proteolytic enzyme and here the most popular is the enzyme from the paw-paw tree called papain. This treatment was patented some 70 years ago in the USA.

With excess polyphenol, the cheapest treatment is addition of formaldehyde to the sweet or hopped wort. But this approach is not permitted in many countries because the formaldehyde reacts with many compounds and may yield some harmful materials. Polyphenolases have been isolated from microorganisms and their use has been advocated on the basis of successes on the pilot-scale.

A further approach is to use absorbents which are insoluble. It is therefore possible to stir them into the lager tank and let them settle after reacting. Alternatively they can be packed into a filter and the beer passed through. The degree of effectiveness will be a function of (among other parameters) the flow of beer through the filter or reactor. Whatever method is employed, the adsorbent does not go into the packaged beer and hence does not have to be admitted as an ingredient. Adsorbents are therefore permitted in West Germany under the beer purity law.

Adsorbents for polyphenols include Nylon 66 and the more recent polymerised polyvinylpyrrolidone (PVPP); both are polyamides and therefore readily form covalent bonds with polyphenols (Fig. 9.4). PVPP can be regenerated from used material by treatment with strong alkali and this fact influences the economics of its use. The important polyphenols in the formation of haze are the dimers (and, possibly, the trimers) of flavone diols. These, when acidified, will yield coloured anthocyanins – flower pigments; they are therefore called anthocyanogens or proanthocyanins.

Turning to the beer proteins, it was a common procedure to treat beer with bentonite, a brick-red earth. This adsorbs the proteins but has two drawbacks; it settles only slowly and its use has an adverse effect on foam stability. A more common adsorbent is silica gel which settles readily and has little effect on foam. The silica gel is manufactured by acidifying sodium silicate under carefully controlled conditions to yield particles of a sponge-like texture and with a huge surface area $(250–1000 \text{ m}^2 \text{ g}^{-1})$. The surface-area-to-volume ratio and the mean pore size can be controlled. Some silica gels are dried by heat to 30% moisture. These are xerogels and contrast with hydrogels where drying (to 70% moisture) also gives a stable product. Particle size, (usually 15–40 μm and controlled by careful milling), determines settling rate in a tank of beer or the effectiveness of action and rate of flow in a packed reactor. The silica gel particles are thought to permit haze-precursor proteins (10000–60000 molecular weight) to enter their pores and be adsorbed. Certainly the preferred pore size is consistent with the molecular size of the precursors. Foam-enhancing glycoproteins probably have a different molecular size and shape and therefore do not enter the pores.

There are many breweries which inject silica gel slurry into the beer line before it reaches the diatomaceous earth (DE, Kieselguhr) filter.

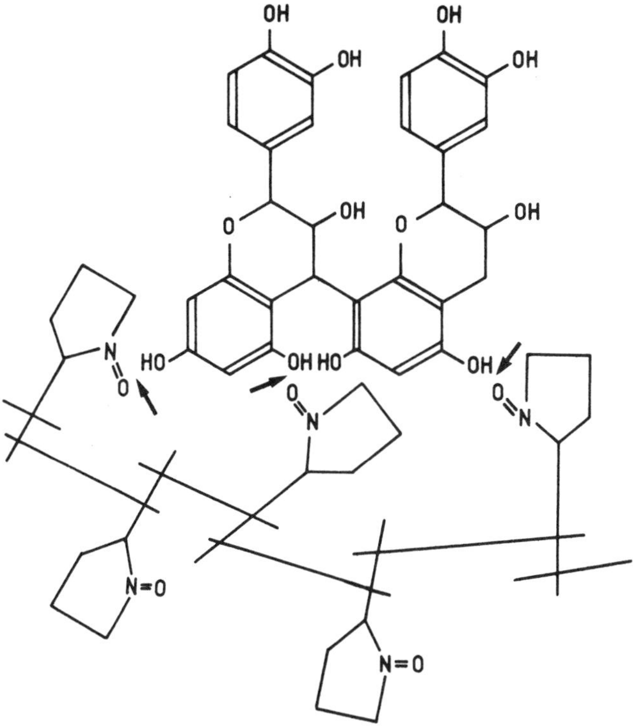

Fig. 9.4. The way in which polyvinylpyrrolidone adsorbs polyphenols.

The silica gel mixes with the DE readily and alters the filtration characteristics very little. It continues to adsorb protein while in the filter. This has been exploited in trial filtrations where DE has been replaced entirely by various grades of silica gel. Both filtration and stabilisation are achieved and the spent material can be used to quench discarded caustic-soda-based detergents. The reason for replacing DE is that it is considered dangerous to the respiratory membranes of workers handling it as a powder.

Filtration

The original filter medium comprised cellulose fibres. They were slurried in water and formed into circular pads that are fitted into a filter frame. Beer passing through the pads has to take a tortuous path in the interstices between the fibres. Suspended particles get trapped at sharp bends and in any cul de sac. As the pad becomes filled with particles, it requires more and more pressure to drive the beer through at the same rate. Back pressure is needed to retain the carbon dioxide in the beer

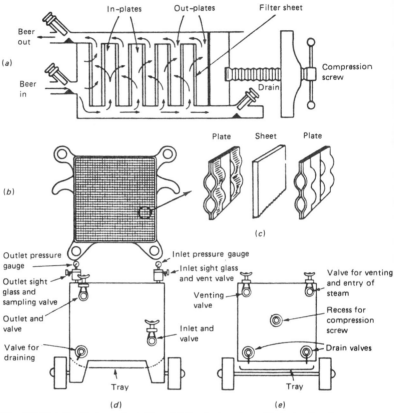

Fig. 9.5. Details of a beer sheet filter. (*a*) Vertical section; (*b*) single plate front view; (*c*) relationship between plates and sheets; (*d*) control end of the machine; (*e*) compression end.

and this too must be compensated for by greater forward pressuring. A maximum of 3 bar pressure above atmospheric is normally imposed. The filter may be back washed to give a limited second life but the pads are then broken up, washed and reconstituted. High manpower costs have greatly reduced the use of this type of filter.

A development using less manpower exploited the filter sheet. Paper and paper board technology was applied to creating a sheet comprising cellulose and asbestos fibres plus Kieselguhr. These rectangular sheets (2.5–5.0 mm thickness), ironed on the side which will face down the process stream, are placed in a filter-frame assembly. Both the principles and operation resemble those of the cellulose pad filter (Fig. 9.5). However, there is the opportunity for the asbestos fibres, because they carry strong positive charges, to attract negatively charged organisms and other suspended particles. Concern about the

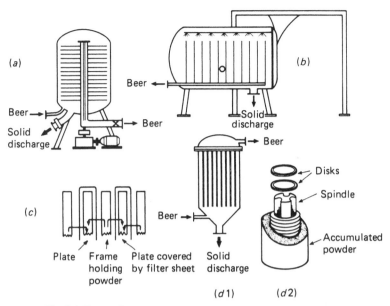

Fig. 9.6. Types of powder filters. (*a*) Vertical sections of a horizontal leaf filter. The motor rotates the spindle and leaves for easy discharge of spent powder. (*b*) Vertical section of a vertical leaf filter. Beer goes in through the central part. The spent powder is washed off by sprays and the leaves can be withdrawn from the filter body. (*c*) Plate and frame filter. Beer moves from frame through powder and sheet before discharge through the plate. (*d*1) Vertical section through a candle filter showing many candles (*d*2) Detail of part of a candle.

carcinogenic properties of asbestos has led to its replacement by other positively charged fibres.

The most popular type of beer filter is the DE or Kieselguhr filter. There are several types (Fig. 9.6) but they all operate on the same principle. Taking the case of the filter leaf assembly, there are perforated or fine-mesh surfaces. These can be coated by coarse Kieselguhr particles pumped through them in the form of a slurry. As the slurry is recycled, the particles bridge the perforations of the leaf (Fig. 9.7) and build up a filter coat. This precoat is usually reinforced by a second, using a finer-grained Kieselguhr. When no Kieselguhr escapes, beer is pumped into the filter. The precoats would soon become blocked with the suspended particles in the beer but this is avoided by regular injections of fresh Kieselguhr into the beer as it enters the filter. This bodyfeed is introduced at just the right concentration to avoid clogging or blinding of the filter medium. Nevertheless it must be used with the utmost economy because eventually the body of the filter becomes entirely filled with Kieselguhr

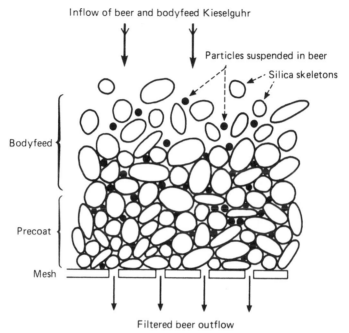

Fig. 9.7. The principle of powder filtration. An initial slurry of powder is made to bridge the holes in the filter leaf. Beer is pumped through, along with regular frequent injections of powder slurry. Suspended particles in the beer become trapped at the interstices between the powder particles.

and filtering then has to cease. Monitoring is partly by forward pressure readings which must not exceed 3 bar above atmospheric; back pressure to retain carbon dioxide in solution is 1 bar. Other monitoring relates to measurement of turbidity and concentration of viable microorganisms.

The candle filter differs from leaf filters insofar as the gaps to be bridged by the Kieselguhr particles are between the edges of circular washers mounted on a hollow central spindle. A candle filter has a vertical cylindrical body enclosing many of these spindle assemblies. With the plate and frame filter, the bodyfeed is coated onto filter sheets which cover hollow plates. The frames accommodate the accumulation of bodyfeed Kieselguhr.

Kieselguhr is an earth that is mined, particularly in Colorado. It comprises the siliceous skeletons of diatoms that lived in seas of the Miocene epoch. The diatoms of many species and shapes sedimented to the sea bottom on death and their skeletons have survived the drying of the seas and their covering with more recent layers of rock. It is necessary to purify the mined material. Heat treatment leads to partial melting of the silica walls and to the gas within expanding to give almost spherical particles (a process which in some ways resembles the making of popcorn). An alternative to Kieselguhr is perlite, a volcanic material mined in certain Greek islands. Both Kieselguhr and perlite are very dusty materials and nowadays great care is taken to avoid the dust coming in contact with workmen, and especially to prevent the powder from being inhaled. The bags are therefore opened with a screen between workmen and the Kieselguhr.

Synthetic polymeric materials have lent themselves to the development of a further type of filter. The simplest is the membrane filter which is a septum perforated with holes whose diameter is carefully controlled to specification. For example one with pores of 1 μm diameter might be expected to prevent yeasts from penetrating, one with pores of 0.2 μm would be expected to hold back bacteria. But these filters will only cope with beer that is virtually free of suspended material. They are therefore only applicable in the process stream after the other types of filter have operated. Their greatest application is in microbiological control. For instance, a sample of bright beer (say 100 ml or even 1 l) is run through a sterilised membrane filter, the filter is then transferred onto the surface of growth medium within a petri dish and incubated. Any colonies developing can be counted and identified. From membrane filters have developed cartridges of pleated membrane with a much greater surface area. The membrane is not uniform; on the upstream surface is a coarse weave of fibres while the downstream surface is similar to a conventional membrane sheet. There is therefore some aspect of depth filtration as in a cellulose/asbestos filter sheet. Such microfibrillar fibres are mainly designed to remove all microorganisms from beer by filtration. Having a similar function is a double filtration system where the second filter comprises fine-grade cellulose/asbestos sheets which remove all microorganisms.

Pasteurisation

The pasteurising of milk is generally familiar but the application of the technique to beer and wine is not. There are two possibilities and both are widely practised. The beer (or wine) may be pasteurised in-line, in other words continuously, by means of a modified heat exchanger (Fig. 9.8). In practice, the beer temperature is raised for a few seconds to about 75 °C. It is, however, difficult to be sure that all the beer actually reaches this temperature. This is not helped by the tendency for carbon dioxide to come out of solution at these temperatures. In order to prevent this occurring, it is necessary to have a forward pressure of about 7.5–10 bar and about 1–5 bar back pressure. Another point is that with many in-line pasteurisers there is a facility for recycling the beer through the equipment when a hold-up occurs. Excessive heat

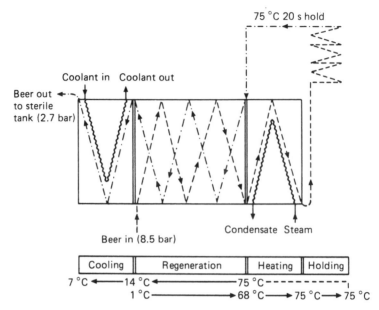

Fig. 9.8. The flow of beer through a continuous or in-line or high-temperature, short-time pasteuriser.

treatment and consequent flavour changes arise. Nevertheless the equipment is compact and not labour-intensive. It is necessary to keep the beer free of infection after treatment and this demands the use of sterilised containers or packages. A further application of this type of equipment is to pasteurise beer returned to the brewery because it is unsatisfactory, beer recovered from filters, yeast pressings and general ullage. Such beer, when pasteurised, is blended into the main stream.

The alternative method is to heat-treat after the beer is in package. This applies particularly to cans of beer and, to some extent, to bottled beer. (In-line equipment can be employed for bottled beer and for beer destined for kegs and bulk delivery.) The cans or bottles are moved progressively through the batch pasteuriser, encountering water sprays of increasing temperature so that the package contents reach 60–5 °C. Cooling sprays then reduce the temperature of the packages before they emerge (Fig. 9.9).

If a typical beer contains a mixed population of common brewery-contaminating bacteria, it can be shown that with temperatures over 50 °C, an increase of 7 deg C accelerates cell kill 10-fold. Furthermore, with a viable population of say 100 cells ml^{-1}, it can be shown that the entire population may be killed by raising the beer temperature to 60 °C for 10 min. The same result will therefore be achieved by the beer temperature being held for 1 min at 65 °C or 6 s at

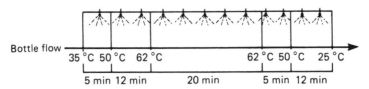

Fig. 9.9. A vertical section through a tunnel pasteuriser.

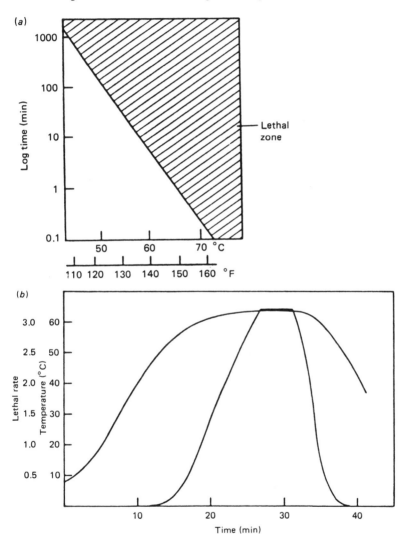

Fig. 9.10. (a) The effect of time and temperature on the viability of a mixed population of yeast and bacterial beer contaminants. The hatched area represents the range of conditions where all the cells are killed. (b) A typical curve (the upper one) for pasteurisation temperatures in a tunnel pasteuriser. The lower curve is the corresponding number of Pasteurisation Units delivered (ordinate 0–3.2). Total Pasteurisation Units is 40.

74 °C for 10 min at 53 °C. For convenience, a Pasteurisation Unit (PU) for beer is defined arbitrarily as the killing effect of holding the beer at 60 °C for 1 min. In a complex treatment (Fig. 9.10), PU are additive. It is therefore possible to compute them from a temperature/time trace or on the basis PU min^{-1} = 1.3^a where a is the relevant temperature (°C) minus 60.

An important consideration is the concentration of viable microoroganisms and their type. The more contaminants that are present, the more is the chance that one or more will survive a heat-treatment. Therefore beer almost free of viable microorganisms (say 1 per 100 ml) is more easily pasteurised than beer with 100 ml^{-1} (Fig. 9.11). However certain wild yeasts and lactic acid bacteria are more heat-resistant than brewing yeasts and acetic acid bacteria. The former thus require more heat treatment to ensure that the beer is effectively pasteurised. In general practice, with less than 100 viable cells per ml, 15–20 PU is suitable for bottles and cans in a batch pasteuriser. In the case of the continuous pasteuriser, it is usual to work at 40–60 PU because there is a greater risk of some of the beer not achieving the specified process temperatures. At these higher PU values, having low dissolved oxygen levels is paramount; otherwise the beer flavour becomes 'cooked', 'biscuity' or 'toast-like'. There may also be greater colour due to oxidation of tannins or melanoidin formation.

One important point is that beer does not normally suffer infections

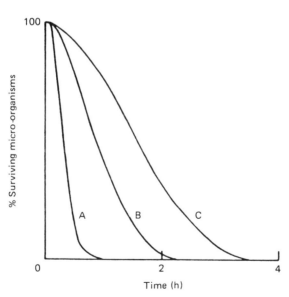

Fig. 9.11. The effect of a killing agent on bacterial populations in beer, A having 100, B with 1000 and C with 100000 cells ml^{-1}.

from spore-forming microorganisms. Spores tend to be more heat-resistant than vegetative cells. Food and beverages that require heat-treatment may be infected with spores which can germinate on those foods. Hence the degree of heat-treatment required may be far more rigorous than that needed for beer. Hence PU for other foods and beverages may be of a greater order of magnitude. However, because beers of low original gravity, low alcohol content and with pH values over 4.4 are subject to mould growth, pasteurisation levels have also to be higher than those for normal beers.

Packaging

Chilled, filtered and continuously pasteurised beer may be transferred to sterilised large tanks (say 8 hl) or kegs (usually 25 or 50 l). Kegs are stainless steel or, more commonly, aluminium containers which differ from traditional casks by having a single opening instead of two. The single opening or neck has screwed into it a device called a spear or extractor. This permits gas (either carbon dioxide or a mixture of 60% nitrogen and 40% carbon dioxide) to be transferred from a gas cylinder to the beer surface. The pressure forces the beer through the base of the extractor tube, up it and out to the pipe connected to the beer dispenser (Fig. 9.12).

Bottles are of two general kinds; those that are used many times and light, less durable one-trip bottles. The multi-trip bottle requires washing, rinsing and draining before it is filled, capped, pasteurised and labelled. One-trip bottles like cans, require only jetting with sterile compressed air and then with sterile water. Some bottles are sterile-filled with beer that has been either continuously pasteurised or sterile-filtered.

The distribution of beer among these various packages varies widely from one country to another. Britain has about 80% of its beer in draught form – in keg, large tank or traditional cask. In the USA, the vast majority of the beer is canned and bottled; in Nigeria it is mainly bottled. Naturally, multi-trip bottles give the heaviest load per hectolitre of beer. Single-trip bottles and cans are much lighter.

Stability

The shelf life of beer depends on a number of factors, but the most important is how quickly the beer will be drunk after packaging. Thus a brewery that can be certain that its beer will be consumed within 1 month does not need to go to the same lengths in stabilising the beer than a brewery whose beer has to keep for a year. Limitations of shelf life are flavour stability, haze stability and microbiological stability.

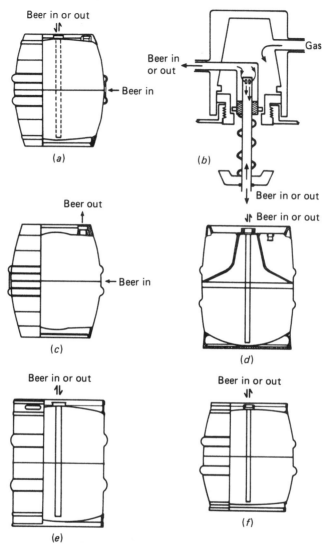

Fig. 9.12. Different types of beer containers. (*a*) Dual-purpose container (for traditional draught ale or for chilled and filtered keg beer). Usually 0.5 or 1.0 hl. (*b*) Section through the fittings of a keg attached to the spear to enable gas to pressurise the beer and cause the beer to rise up the spear. (*c*) A traditional draught cask – may be 18, 36 or 54 gallon or 0.5 or 1.0 hl. (*d*) Keg with in-built gas chamber. (*e*) Straight-sided 0.5 hl keg. (*f*) Barrel-shaped keg – sizes as for (*c*).

Dissolved oxygen is the most important factor because it seriously affects each of these three types of stability. It must therefore be kept to a low level (say below 0.3 ppm) in the packaged beer where long shelf life is required. Another important factor is temperature. One large US brewery ensures that all beer is kept chilled from fermentor to the supermarket shelves; it receives no pasteurisation. At low temperatures there is less chance of deterioration with respect to flavour, haze or infection.

Beer composition

Beer comprises over 400 different compounds in addition to the macromolecular proteins, nucleic acids, carbohydrates and lipids. Some are derived from raw materials and are unchanged through the brewing process, others are radically changed. The most abundant constituent of beer is water and other simple substances include a variety of ions and carbon dioxide (3.5–6.5 g/l). Ethanol levels vary greatly but with most beers produced in the world of OG 1042–4, they are often 3.6–4.2% (v/v).

The spectrum of carbohydrates is greatly influenced by the use of amyloglucosidase preparations in the fermentor. Expressed in terms of glucose, those so treated have 0.4–0.9% (w/v) and traditional beers have 0.9–3.0% (w/v). Unless fermentation has been incomplete or sugars added in excess after fermentation, the most important carbohydrates will be dextrins and fermentable sugars will be in trace amounts.

Non-volatile constituents will include glycerol from yeast metabolism (1.5–3.5 g l^{-1}), lipids (0.5 mg l^{-1}) and the larger fatty acids (0.5 mg l^{-1}). Polyphenols account for some 80–160 mg l^{-1} and hop bitter resins for 30–40 mg l^{-1}. Nitrogenous compounds are in the region 300–900 mg N l^{-1} and comprise denatured proteins, denatured nucleic acid, amino acids, amides, amines and heterocyclic compounds. Volatile compounds, besides ethanol, will include alcohols of greater molecular size (100–200 mg l^{-1}), esters (25–40 mg l^{-1}), acids (say 15 mg l^{-1}), aldehydes (say 48 mg l^{-1}), and ketones (say 3 mg l^{-1}). Strongly aromatic compounds such as diacetyl may be in the range 0.1–2 mg l^{-1} but dimethyl sulphide levels would be only 15–150 μg l^{-1} (Table 9.1).

The calorific value of beer is mainly derived from ethanol, residual carbohydrate and protein. It is calculated in Kcal per 100 ml by multiplying the beer solids (as % w/v) by four and adding to it seven times the ethanol content (as % w/v). Beer also contains B group vitamins such as biotin, nicotinic acid, pantothenic acid, pyridoxine, riboflavin, thiamine, folic acid and vitamin B_{12}. A litre of beer may therefore provide 300–400 Kcal (or 1200–1600 kJ), 3 g 'protein' and

Table 9.1. *Some flavour and aroma compounds associated with yeast metabolism*

Class of Volatile	Name	Taste threshold in degassed beer (ppm)	Content in ale (ppm)	Content in lager (ppm)	Content in stout (ppm)
Alcohols	Ethanol	—	$27-32 \times 10^3$	24×10^3	$16-72 \times 10^3$
	Isopentanol	50	47-61	32-57	33-169
	B phenyl ethanol	50	36-53	25-32	20-55
	n-propanol	50	31-48	5-10	13-60
	Isobutanol	100	18-33	6-11	11-98
	2-methyl butanol	50	14-19	8-16	9-41
Esters	Ethyl acetate	5	14-23	8-14	11-69
	Isopentyl acetate	1	1.4-3.3	1.5-2.0	1.0-4.9
Diketone	Diacetyl[a]	0.005	0.06-0.30	0.02-0.08	0.02-0.07
	Pentane-2,3-dione	—	0.01-0.20	0.01-0.05	0.01-0.08
Sulphur compounds	Hydrogen sulphide[a]	0.005-0.010	0.0015-0.008	0.0015-0.008	0.0015-0.008
	Dimethyl sulphide[a]	33 (ppb)	15+ (ppb)	15+ (ppb)	15+ (ppb)

[a] In beer some may be derived from bacteria present during fermentation.

some contribution of vitamin B. However some 4 l of beer would be needed to provide the daily riboflavin requirement and about 20 l of beer to furnish the total daily need for protein. Beer is therefore a calorie-rich beverage but certainly not a balanced food.

Beer quality

There was a time when one brewery could successfully market its product by the slogan 'G____ is good for you'. While this slogan was true then and now, the customer is also concerned with flavour, aroma, colour, foam and presentation. The beverage appeals in many senses. A customer may be attracted to it by seeing it in a glass with a rich creamy foam. When brought to the lips, the aroma of the beer may excite the olfactory senses. As the beer passes over the tongue and back of the mouth, the various taste-buds will be stimulated by the complex flavour (Table 9.2). Volatiles will diffuse into the back of the nose. Finally, the alcohol is quickly absorbed into the bloodstream and gives a sense of mild euphoria.

The brewer must formulate and brew to arrive at a product that will appeal to as large a group of customers as possible. Having achieved success, the brewer must attempt to maintain the characteristics of the beer, despite some variation in the raw materials. He has to measure certain parameters that will give him the simplest possible 'fingerprint'. The measurements may be analytical such as specific gravity, colour, ethanol content and so on, but these must be supplemented by flavour and aroma assessments.

There are many problems associated with such assessments. Language presents a difficulty, for instance people may differ in their understanding of the expression 'hoppy taste' or 'vegetable flavour' or 'spicy aroma'. With laboratory personnel, even general brewery staff, it is possible to train panels using a library of pure compounds or

Table 9.2. *Partial summary of some human taste sensations*

Sensation	Locus	Stimuli	Receptor	Ganglion
Salty	Anterior tongue, palate	NaCl, KCl	Taste buds	Geniculate
Sour	Anterior tongue, palate	Malic acid	Taste buds	Geniculate
Sweet$_1$	Anterior tongue, palate	L-Alanine, fructose	Taste buds	Geniculate
Bitter$_1$	Anterior tongue, palate	L-Tryptophan	Taste buds	Geniculate
Pleasant	Anterior tongue, palate	Lactones	Taste buds	Geniculate
Sweet$_2$	Posterior tongue	Dihydrochalcone	Taste buds	Petrous
Bitter$_2$	Posterior tongue	$MgSO_4$ phenolics	Taste buds	Petrous
Astringent	Oral cavity	Theaflavin	Free nerve	Trigeminal
Pungent	Oral cavity	Capsaicin	Free nerve	Trigeminal
Metallic	Tongue	Silver nitrate	Taste buds(?)	Petrous

complex preparations so that all are able to identify certain named flavours or aromas. But the trained brewery workers are not necessarily representative of the customers. Furthermore, laboratory conditions for taste testing may be a far cry from the relaxed atmosphere of the home or pub bar. Hence there has emerged a distinction between the panels in the brewery that have an analytical role and informal gatherings of potential or actual customers whose purpose is to indicate approval or otherwise in as quantitative a fashion as is realistic.

Laboratory taste panels may be used to select able judges of beer, to correlate taste assessments with chemical or physical measurements, to monitor the beer from brew to brew and to assess changes in raw materials or processing. Many different tests may be used and only a small selection of these will be described. They include difference tests, ranking-in-order tests, scoring tests, descriptive tests and acceptance or preference tests.

Difference tests are often carried out most effectively by teenagers who do not smoke and who do not drink heavily; girls tend to perform better than boys in the tests. The test may be between two beers – are they different? Alternatively three beers may be presented – which is the odd one or which represent a matched pair? With the two-glass test, there is a 50% possibility of being correct by chance, with the three-glass test there is a 33.3% chance. Statistical tables indicate that with a panel of 20 tasters, if 15 are correct in a two-glass test or 11 in a three-glass test, there is a 5% possibility that the result has been arrived at by chance rather than skill. For 0.1% possibility of chance, the corresponding number of correct answers is 18 and 14 respectively. The panel should be housed comfortably, free from noise or odour, with the beer in identical glasses which should be opaque (or the room darkened). Naturally the answer is only disclosed after all the panel has completed the test.

With a trained panel, a list of flavour and aroma attributes may be listed on sheets given to each taster. The panelist may indicate intensity by a number (say from 1, which is equivalent to slight, through to 5, which is extreme). Total scores can then be assembled. Indeed extremely complicated mathematics may now be introduced using a computer as the instrument to handle the numbers. One technique is discriminant or cluster analysis. Here each parameter measured represents a dimension, so that if 20 parameters are involved, there are 20 dimensions. A beer is represented by a point in this multi-dimensional space. Beers similar to it will tend to be close to it but beers very different are remote from it in the space. A computer programme can now be exploited that transforms this multi-dimensional space into a two-dimensional display (Fig. 9.13). The axes are mathematical abstractions but nevertheless very convenient for easy visualisation.

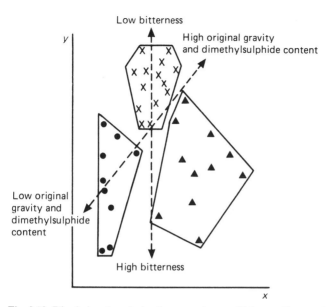

Fig. 9.13. Discriminant analysis of sensory data on 33 lagers. Crosses: North American lagers; circles: British lagers; and triangles: continental European lagers. Arrows indicate the general movements with respect to bitterness, dimethyl sulphide content and original gravity. The coordinates are mathematical abstractions to bring 27-dimensional space into terms of two dimensions.

A further consideration is preference tasting and this may be added to the two-glass or three-glass tasting routine or to the more complex tests described above. Breweries differ greatly in the way in which they carry out taste-testing and evaluations but one of the most comprehensive schemes has been devised by a large brewery in the USA. It has a permanent trained panel in the brewery and creates *ad hoc* panels both from brewery visitors and from groups of people who chance to meet at trade conventions or social functions. The trained panel use a form of the discriminant analysis based on some 10 attributes of beer that are considered paramount. (They include sulphury aroma, after-taste, bitterness, metallic flavour, caramel, sweet, fruity aroma, 'body of the beer', and carbonation.) Comparisons are made between beers produced by the company and those that are current market leaders. Changes are made to the characters of the beer under scrutiny, by altering raw materials and/or processing, to make it close to the market leader or to satisfy the preferences expressed by the lay panels. The method can also be used to bring each beer brand of various breweries in a company closer together. It also has the potential, although this will be expensive, of carrying out an evaluation of raw materials and steps in processing. This would indicate the tolerances that are acceptable in these areas.

There are of course major problems. The preferences of the public change over a period of time and are readily swayed by advertising. Between 1960 and 1980, several UK city breweries experienced a swing from the dark, sweet, less hopped, draught mild beers to pale, draught bitter beers. The proportions of mild to pale changed in some instances from 5:1 to 1:5. Over the past 10 years, lager beer in the UK has increased its share of the market substantially and now represents some 30% of the total. Still another swing in Britain is the increasing preference for fruit-based drinks such as cider and wine over beers. In other countries, such as Spain and Nigeria, the trend is in the opposite direction.

One other development in the UK and USA has been the growth over the past 10 years or more of very small breweries producing distinctive products and each employing no more than a handful of people. There is too an increasing band of people who brew at home not only because they produce their beer cheaply but also because the making of it provides a pastime. A small industry has grown supplying special hopped extracts and other requirements for the home-brewers. Brewing as a whole therefore spans from high technology with microprocessors to the hobby at home. One fascinating point is that, whatever the scale, the biological, biochemical, chemical and physical principles are the same.

Further Reading

1. J. S. Hough, D. E. Briggs, R. Stevens & T. W. Young (1982). *Malting and Brewing Science* (2 volumes), London: Chapman & Hall.
2. D. E. Briggs (1978). *Barley*, London: Chapman & Hall.
3. H. M. Broderick (ed.) (1977). *The Practical Brewer*. Madison, Wisconsin: Master Brewers Association of the Americas.
4. J. R. A. Pollock (ed.) (1979 and subsequently). *Brewing Science* (3 volumes). London & New York: Academic Press.

Conversions

Weight

Metric ton = 2204.6 lb

kg = 2.205 lb

SI units are kg, g, mg, μg

    Zentner (hops) = 50 kg (110.2 lb)

    Qr (barley) = 448 lb

    Qr (malt) = 336 lb

US & Canadian

    bushel (barley) = 48 lb

US & Canadian

    bushel (malt) = 34 lb

Imperial (long) ton = 2240 lb

cwt = 112 lb

lb = 0.454 lb

oz = 28.35 g

grain = 64.80 mg

Volume

cubic metre = 33.315 cu ft

cubic metre = 219.98 British gallon

cubic metre = 264.18 US gallon

cubic metre = 10 hl

cubic metre = 1000 l

British barrel = 36 British gallon

US barrel = 31 US gallon

US barrel = 1.1734 hl

Butt = 108 British gallon

Hogshead = 54 British gallon

Barrel = 36 British gallon

Kilderkin = 18 British gallon

Firkin = 9 British gallon

Pin = 4.5 British gallon

British gallon = 8 pints

British gallon = 160 fluid oz

British gallon = 454.6 cl

Ratios

1 lb per gallon (British) = 99.76 g/l^{-1}

1 lb per barrel (British) = 2.77 g l^{-1}

1 grain per gallon

    (British) = 14.25 mg l^{-1}

1 oz per gallon (British) = 623.6 g l^{-1}

100% proof spirit = 57.10% alcohol

by volume = 49.28% by weight

1 g CO_2 per 100 ml beer = 5.06

volumes

Index